ACCESS YOUR ONLINE RESOURCES

AF598769

DON'T MISS OUT ON THE ONLINE RESOURCES INCLUDED WITH YOUR PURCHASE!

Your purchase of this product unlocks access to our Online Resources page. Elevate your study experience with our **interactive practice test interface**, along with all of the additional resources that we couldn't include in this book.

Flip to the Online Resources section at the end of this book to find the link and a QR code to get started!

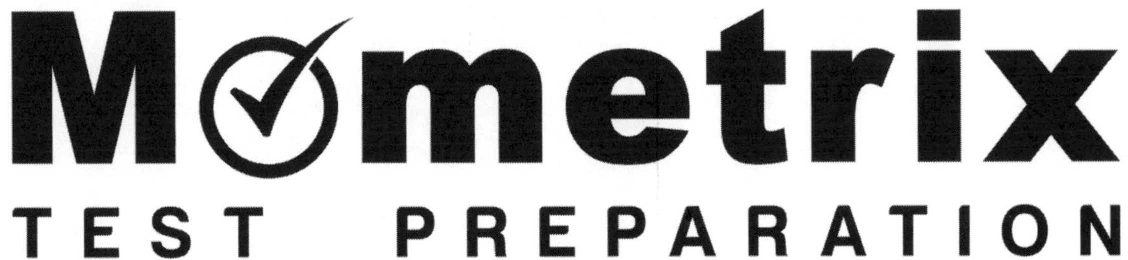

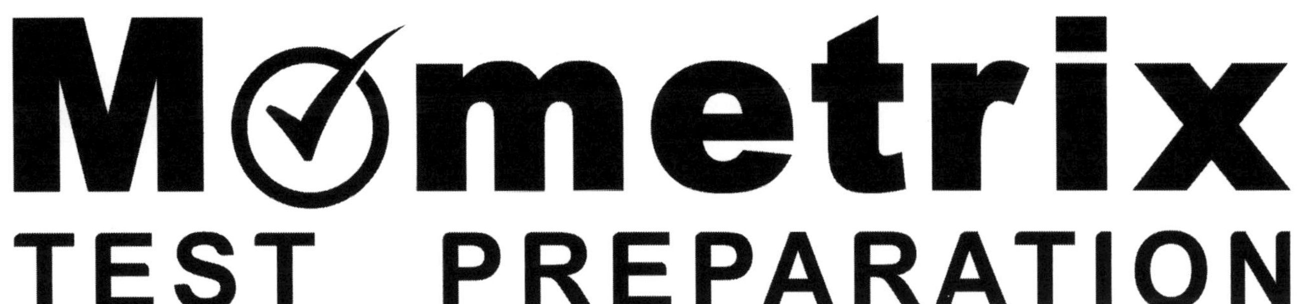

ACHPN®

Exam Secrets Study Guide

Unofficial ACHPN® Test Review for the Advanced Certified Hospice and Palliative Nurse Examination

Written and edited by Mometrix Test Prep

Printed in the United States of America

This paper meets the requirements of ANSI/NISO Z39.48-1992 (Permanence of Paper).

Paperback
ISBN 13: 978-1-5167-0875-8
ISBN 10: 1-5167-0875-X

Dear Future Exam Success Story

First of all, **THANK YOU** for purchasing Mometrix study materials!

Second, congratulations! You are one of the few determined test-takers who are committed to doing whatever it takes to excel on your exam. **You have come to the right place.** We developed these study materials with one goal in mind: to deliver you the information you need in a format that's concise and easy to use.

In addition to optimizing your guide for the content of the test, we've outlined our recommended steps for breaking down the preparation process into small, attainable goals so you can make sure you stay on track.

We've also analyzed the entire test-taking process, identifying the most common pitfalls and showing how you can overcome them and be ready for any curveball the test throws you.

Standardized testing is one of the biggest obstacles on your road to success, which only increases the importance of doing well in the high-pressure, high-stakes environment of test day. Your results on this test could have a significant impact on your future, and this guide provides the information and practical advice to help you achieve your full potential on test day.

Your success is our success

We would love to hear from you! If you would like to share the story of your exam success or if you have any questions or comments in regard to our products, please contact us at **800-673-8175** or **support@mometrix.com**.

Thanks again for your business and we wish you continued success!

Sincerely,
The Mometrix Test Preparation Team

Need more help? Check out our flashcards at:
http://mometrixflashcards.com/NBCHPN

Written and edited by the Mometrix Exam Secrets Test Prep Team
Printed in the United States of America

TABLE OF CONTENTS

Introduction

Thank you for purchasing this resource! You have made the choice to prepare yourself for a test that could have a huge impact on your future, and this guide is designed to help you be fully ready for test day. Obviously, it's important to have a solid understanding of the test material, but you also need to be prepared for the unique environment and stressors of the test, so that you can perform to the best of your abilities.

For this purpose, the first section that appears in this guide is the **Secret Keys**. We've devoted countless hours to meticulously researching what works and what doesn't, and we've boiled down our findings to the five most impactful steps you can take to improve your performance on the test. We start at the beginning with study planning and move through the preparation process, all the way to the testing strategies that will help you get the most out of what you know when you're finally sitting in front of the test.

We recommend that you start preparing for your test as far in advance as possible. However, if you've bought this guide as a last-minute study resource and only have a few days before your test, we recommend that you skip over the first two Secret Keys since they address a long-term study plan.

If you struggle with **test anxiety**, we strongly encourage you to check out our recommendations for how you can overcome it. Test anxiety is a formidable foe, but it can be beaten, and we want to make sure you have the tools you need to defeat it.

Secret Key #1 – Plan Big, Study Small

There's a lot riding on your performance. If you want to ace this test, you're going to need to keep your skills sharp and the material fresh in your mind. You need a plan that lets you review everything you need to know while still fitting in your schedule. We'll break this strategy down into three categories.

Information Organization

Start with the information you already have: the official test outline. From this, you can make a complete list of all the concepts you need to cover before the test. Organize these concepts into groups that can be studied together, and create a list of any related vocabulary you need to learn so you can brush up on any difficult terms. You'll want to keep this vocabulary list handy once you actually start studying since you may need to add to it along the way.

Time Management

Once you have your set of study concepts, decide how to spread them out over the time you have left before the test. Break your study plan into small, clear goals so you have a manageable task for each day and know exactly what you're doing. Then just focus on one small step at a time. When you manage your time this way, you don't need to spend hours at a time studying. Studying a small block of content for a short period each day helps you retain information better and avoid stressing over how much you have left to do. You can relax knowing that you have a plan to cover everything in time. In order for this strategy to be effective though, you have to start studying early and stick to your schedule. Avoid the exhaustion and futility that comes from last-minute cramming!

Study Environment

The environment you study in has a big impact on your learning. Studying in a coffee shop, while probably more enjoyable, is not likely to be as fruitful as studying in a quiet room. It's important to keep distractions to a minimum. You're only planning to study for a short block of time, so make the most of it. Don't pause to check your phone or get up to find a snack. It's also important to **avoid multitasking**. Research has consistently shown that multitasking will make your studying dramatically less effective. Your study area should also be comfortable and well-lit so you don't have the distraction of straining your eyes or sitting on an uncomfortable chair.

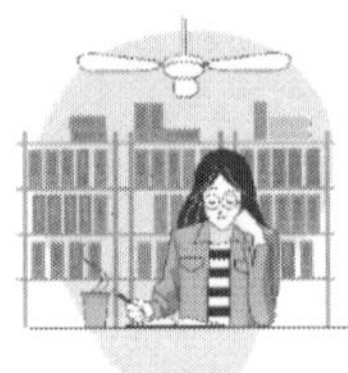

The time of day you study is also important. You want to be rested and alert. Don't wait until just before bedtime. Study when you'll be most likely to comprehend and remember. Even better, if you know what time of day your test will be, set that time aside for study. That way your brain will be used to working on that subject at that specific time and you'll have a better chance of recalling information.

Finally, it can be helpful to team up with others who are studying for the same test. Your actual studying should be done in as isolated an environment as possible, but the work of organizing the information and setting up the study plan can be divided up. In between study sessions, you can discuss with your teammates the concepts that you're all studying and quiz each other on the details. Just be sure that your teammates are as serious about the test as you are. If you find that your study time is being replaced with social time, you might need to find a new team.

Secret Key #2 – Make Your Studying Count

You're devoting a lot of time and effort to preparing for this test, so you want to be absolutely certain it will pay off. This means doing more than just reading the content and hoping you can remember it on test day. It's important to make every minute of study count. There are two main areas you can focus on to make your studying count.

Retention

It doesn't matter how much time you study if you can't remember the material. You need to make sure you are retaining the concepts. To check your retention of the information you're learning, try recalling it at later times with minimal prompting. Try carrying around flashcards and glance at one or two from time to time or ask a friend who's also studying for the test to quiz you.

To enhance your retention, look for ways to put the information into practice so that you can apply it rather than simply recalling it. If you're using the information in practical ways, it will be much easier to remember. Similarly, it helps to solidify a concept in your mind if you're not only reading it to yourself but also explaining it to someone else. Ask a friend to let you teach them about a concept you're a little shaky on (or speak aloud to an imaginary audience if necessary). As you try to summarize, define, give examples, and answer your friend's questions, you'll understand the concepts better and they will stay with you longer. Finally, step back for a big picture view and ask yourself how each piece of information fits with the whole subject. When you link the different concepts together and see them working together as a whole, it's easier to remember the individual components.

Finally, practice showing your work on any multi-step problems, even if you're just studying. Writing out each step you take to solve a problem will help solidify the process in your mind, and you'll be more likely to remember it during the test.

Modality

Modality simply refers to the means or method by which you study. Choosing a study modality that fits your own individual learning style is crucial. No two people learn best in exactly the same way, so it's important to know your strengths and use them to your advantage.

For example, if you learn best by visualization, focus on visualizing a concept in your mind and draw an image or a diagram. Try color-coding your notes, illustrating them, or creating symbols that will trigger your mind to recall a learned concept. If you learn best by hearing or discussing information, find a study partner who learns the same way or read aloud to yourself. Think about how to put the information in your own words. Imagine that you are giving a lecture on the topic and record yourself so you can listen to it later.

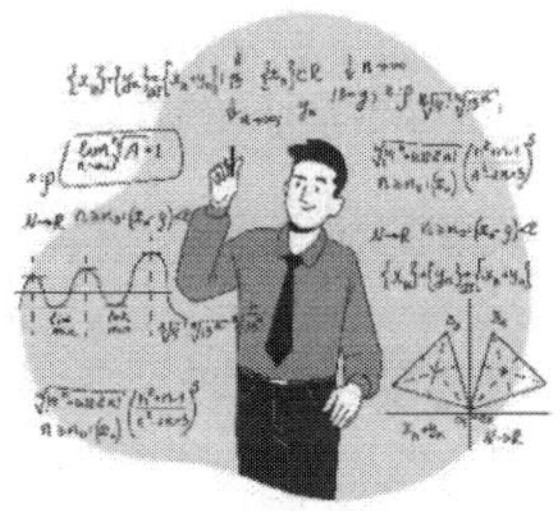

For any learning style, flashcards can be helpful. Organize the information so you can take advantage of spare moments to review. Underline key words or phrases. Use different colors for different categories. Mnemonic devices (such as creating a short list in which every item starts with the same letter) can also help with retention. Find what works best for you and use it to store the information in your mind most effectively and easily.

Secret Key #3 – Practice the Right Way

Your success on test day depends not only on how many hours you put into preparing, but also on whether you prepared the right way. It's good to check along the way to see if your studying is paying off. One of the most effective ways to do this is by taking practice tests to evaluate your progress. Practice tests are useful because they show exactly where you need to improve. Every time you take a practice test, pay special attention to these three groups of questions:

- The questions you got wrong
- The questions you had to guess on, even if you guessed right
- The questions you found difficult or slow to work through

This will show you exactly what your weak areas are, and where you need to devote more study time. Ask yourself why each of these questions gave you trouble. Was it because you didn't understand the material? Was it because you didn't remember the vocabulary? Do you need more repetitions on this type of question to build speed and confidence? Dig into those questions and figure out how you can strengthen your weak areas as you go back to review the material.

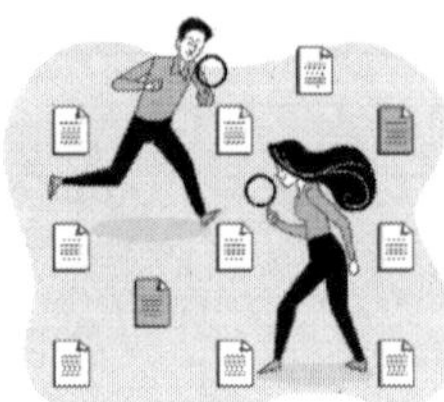

Additionally, many practice tests have a section explaining the answer choices. It can be tempting to read the explanation and think that you now have a good understanding of the concept. However, an explanation likely only covers part of the question's broader context. Even if the explanation makes perfect sense, **go back and investigate** every concept related to the question until you're positive you have a thorough understanding.

As you go along, keep in mind that the practice test is just that: practice. Memorizing these questions and answers will not be very helpful on the actual test because it is unlikely to have any of the same exact questions. If you only know the right answers to the sample questions, you won't be prepared for the real thing. **Study the concepts** until you understand them fully, and then you'll be able to answer any question that shows up on the test.

It's important to wait on the practice tests until you're ready. If you take a test on your first day of study, you may be overwhelmed by the amount of material covered and how much you need to learn. Work up to it gradually.

On test day, you'll need to be prepared for answering questions, managing your time, and using the test-taking strategies you've learned. It's a lot to balance, like a mental marathon that will have a big impact on your future. Like training for a marathon, you'll need to start slowly and work your way up. When test day arrives, you'll be ready.

Start with the strategies you've read in the first two Secret Keys—plan your course and study in the way that works best for you. If you have time, consider using multiple study resources to get different approaches to the same concepts. It can be helpful to see difficult concepts from more than one angle. Then find a good source for practice tests. Many times, the test website will suggest potential study resources or provide sample tests.

Practice Test Strategy

If you're able to find at least three practice tests, we recommend this strategy:

Untimed and Open-Book Practice

Take the first test with no time constraints and with your notes and study guide handy. Take your time and focus on applying the strategies you've learned.

Timed and Open-Book Practice

Take the second practice test open-book as well, but set a timer and practice pacing yourself to finish in time.

Timed and Closed-Book Practice

Take any other practice tests as if it were test day. Set a timer and put away your study materials. Sit at a table or desk in a quiet room, imagine yourself at the testing center, and answer questions as quickly and accurately as possible.

Keep repeating timed and closed-book tests on a regular basis until you run out of practice tests or it's time for the actual test. Your mind will be ready for the schedule and stress of test day, and you'll be able to focus on recalling the material you've learned.

Secret Key #4 – Pace Yourself

Once you're fully prepared for the material on the test, your biggest challenge on test day will be managing your time. Just knowing that the clock is ticking can make you panic even if you have plenty of time left. Work on pacing yourself so you can build confidence against the time constraints of the exam. Pacing is a difficult skill to master, especially in a high-pressure environment, so **practice is vital**.

Set time expectations for your pace based on how much time is available. For example, if a section has 60 questions and the time limit is 30 minutes, you know you have to average 30 seconds or less per question in order to answer them all. Although 30 seconds is the hard limit, set 25 seconds per question as your goal, so you reserve extra time to spend on harder questions. When you budget extra time for the harder questions, you no longer have any reason to stress when those questions take longer to answer.

Don't let this time expectation distract you from working through the test at a calm, steady pace, but keep it in mind so you don't spend too much time on any one question. Recognize that taking extra time on one question you don't understand may keep you from answering two that you do understand later in the test. If your time limit for a question is up and you're still not sure of the answer, mark it and move on, and come back to it later if the time and the test format allow. If the testing format doesn't allow you to return to earlier questions, just make an educated guess; then put it out of your mind and move on.

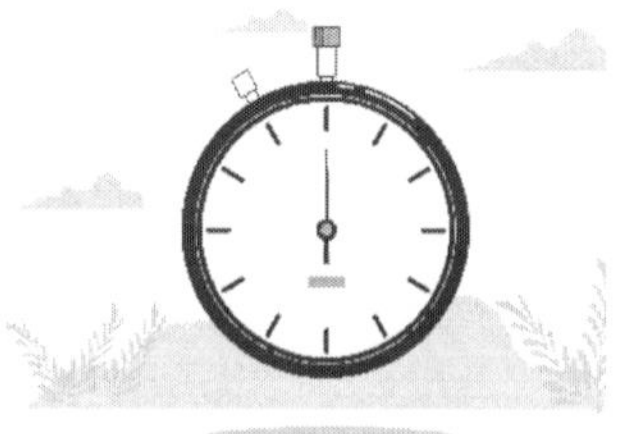

On the easier questions, be careful not to rush. It may seem wise to hurry through them so you have more time for the challenging ones, but it's not worth missing one if you know the concept and just didn't take the time to read the question fully. Work efficiently but make sure you understand the question and have looked at all of the answer choices, since more than one may seem right at first.

Even if you're paying attention to the time, you may find yourself a little behind at some point. You should speed up to get back on track, but do so wisely. Don't panic; just take a few seconds less on each question until you're caught up. Don't guess without thinking, but do look through the answer choices and eliminate any you know are wrong. If you can get down to two choices, it is often worthwhile to guess from those. Once you've chosen an answer, move on and don't dwell on any that you skipped or had to hurry through. If a question was taking too long, chances are it was one of the harder ones, so you weren't as likely to get it right anyway.

On the other hand, if you find yourself getting ahead of schedule, it may be beneficial to slow down a little. The more quickly you work, the more likely you are to make a careless mistake that will affect your score. You've budgeted time for each question, so don't be afraid to spend that time. Practice an efficient but careful pace to get the most out of the time you have.

Secret Key #5 – Have a Plan for Guessing

When you're taking the test, you may find yourself stuck on a question. Some of the answer choices seem better than others, but you don't see the one answer choice that is obviously correct. What do you do?

The scenario described above is very common, yet most test takers have not effectively prepared for it. Developing and practicing a plan for guessing may be one of the single most effective uses of your time as you get ready for the exam.

In developing your plan for guessing, there are three questions to address:

- When should you start the guessing process?
- How should you narrow down the choices?
- Which answer should you choose?

When to Start the Guessing Process

Unless your plan for guessing is to select C every time (which, despite its merits, is not what we recommend), you need to leave yourself enough time to apply your answer elimination strategies. Since you have a limited amount of time for each question, that means that if you're going to give yourself the best shot at guessing correctly, you have to decide quickly whether or not you will guess.

Of course, the best-case scenario is that you don't have to guess at all, so first, see if you can answer the question based on your knowledge of the subject and basic reasoning skills. Focus on the key words in the question and try to jog your memory of related topics. Give yourself a chance to bring the knowledge to mind, but once you realize that you don't have (or you can't access) the knowledge you need to answer the question, it's time to start the guessing process.

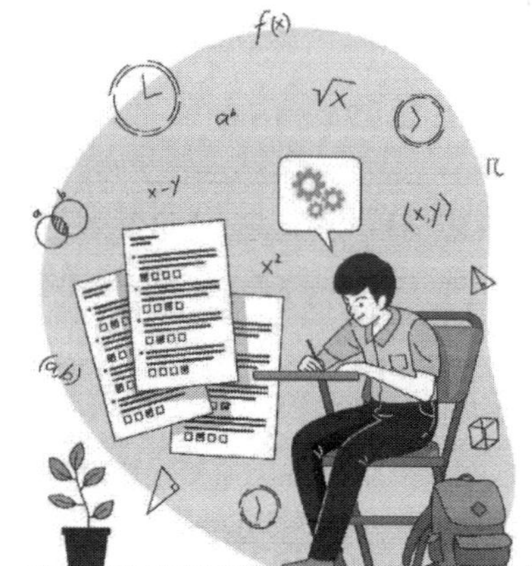

It's almost always better to start the guessing process too early than too late. It only takes a few seconds to remember something and answer the question from knowledge. Carefully eliminating wrong answer choices takes longer. Plus, going through the process of eliminating answer choices can actually help jog your memory.

Summary: Start the guessing process as soon as you decide that you can't answer the question based on your knowledge.

How to Narrow Down the Choices

The next chapter in this book (**Test-Taking Strategies**) includes a wide range of strategies for how to approach questions and how to look for answer choices to eliminate. You will definitely want to read those carefully, practice them, and figure out which ones work best for you. Here though, we're going to address a mindset rather than a particular strategy.

Your odds of guessing an answer correctly depend on how many options you are choosing from.

Number of options left	5	4	3	2	1
Odds of guessing correctly	20%	25%	33%	50%	100%

You can see from this chart just how valuable it is to be able to eliminate incorrect answers and make an educated guess, but there are two things that many test takers do that cause them to miss out on the benefits of guessing:

- Accidentally eliminating the correct answer
- Selecting an answer based on an impression

We'll look at the first one here, and the second one in the next section.

To avoid accidentally eliminating the correct answer, we recommend a thought exercise called **the $5 challenge**. In this challenge, you only eliminate an answer choice from contention if you are willing to bet $5 on it being wrong. Why $5? Five dollars is a small but not insignificant amount of money. It's an amount you could afford to lose but wouldn't want to throw away. And while losing $5 once might not hurt too much, doing it twenty times will set you back $100. In the same way, each small decision you make—eliminating a choice here, guessing on a question there—won't by itself impact your score very much, but when you put them all together, they can make a big difference. By holding each answer choice elimination decision to a higher standard, you can reduce the risk of accidentally eliminating the correct answer.

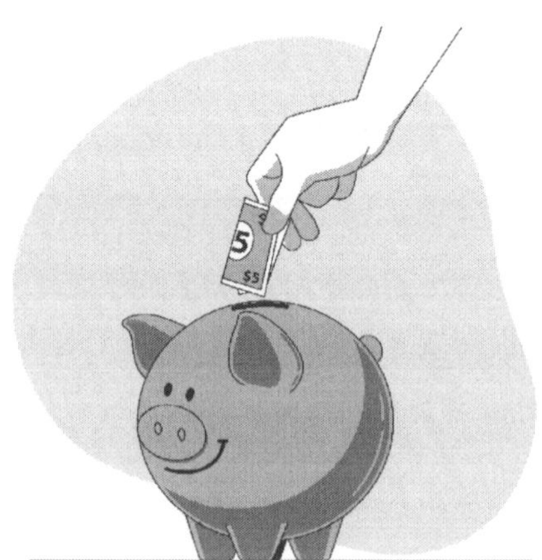

The $5 challenge can also be applied in a positive sense: If you are willing to bet $5 that an answer choice *is* correct, go ahead and mark it as correct.

Summary: Only eliminate an answer choice if you are willing to bet $5 that it is wrong.

Which Answer to Choose

You're taking the test. You've run into a hard question and decided you'll have to guess. You've eliminated all the answer choices you're willing to bet $5 on. Now you have to pick an answer. Why do we even need to talk about this? Why can't you just pick whichever one you feel like when the time comes?

The answer to these questions is that if you don't come into the test with a plan, you'll rely on your impression to select an answer choice, and if you do that, you risk falling into a trap. The test writers know that everyone who takes their test will be guessing on some of the questions, so they intentionally write wrong answer choices to seem plausible. You still have to pick an answer though, and if the wrong answer choices are designed to look right, how can you ever be sure that you're not falling for their trap? The best solution we've found to this dilemma is to take the decision out of your hands entirely. Here is the process we recommend:

Once you've eliminated any choices that you are confident (willing to bet $5) are wrong, select the first remaining choice as your answer.

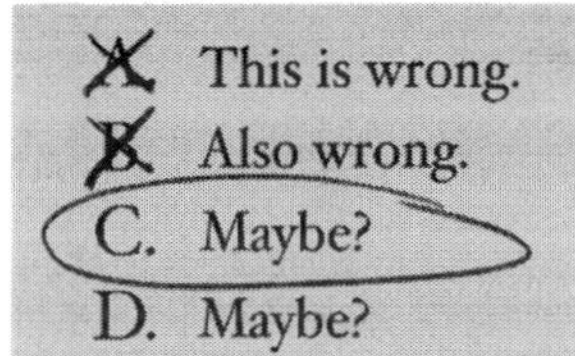

Whether you choose to select the first remaining choice, the second, or the last, the important thing is that you use some preselected standard. Using this approach guarantees that you will not be enticed into selecting an answer choice that looks right, because you are not basing your decision on how the answer choices look.

This is not meant to make you question your knowledge. Instead, it is to help you recognize the difference between your knowledge and your impressions. There's a huge difference between thinking an answer is right because of what you know, and thinking an answer is right because it looks or sounds like it should be right.

Summary: To ensure that your selection is appropriately random, make a predetermined selection from among all answer choices you have not eliminated.

Test-Taking Strategies

This section contains a list of test-taking strategies that you may find helpful as you work through the test. By taking what you know and applying logical thought, you can maximize your chances of answering any question correctly!

It is very important to realize that every question is different and every person is different: no single strategy will work on every question, and no single strategy will work for every person. That's why we've included all of them here, so you can try them out and determine which ones work best for different types of questions and which ones work best for you.

Question Strategies

✓ Read Carefully

Read the question and the answer choices carefully. Don't miss the question because you misread the terms. You have plenty of time to read each question thoroughly and make sure you understand what is being asked. Yet a happy medium must be attained, so don't waste too much time. You must read carefully and efficiently.

✓ Contextual Clues

Look for contextual clues. If the question includes a word you are not familiar with, look at the immediate context for some indication of what the word might mean. Contextual clues can often give you all the information you need to decipher the meaning of an unfamiliar word. Even if you can't determine the meaning, you may be able to narrow down the possibilities enough to make a solid guess at the answer to the question.

✓ Prefixes

If you're having trouble with a word in the question or answer choices, try dissecting it. Take advantage of every clue that the word might include. Prefixes can be a huge help. Usually, they allow you to determine a basic meaning. *Pre-* means before, *post-* means after, *pro-* is positive, *de-* is negative. From prefixes, you can get an idea of the general meaning of the word and try to put it into context.

✓ Hedge Words

Watch out for critical hedge words, such as *likely, may, can, often, almost, mostly, usually, generally, rarely,* and *sometimes.* Question writers insert these hedge phrases to cover every possibility. Often an answer choice will be wrong simply because it leaves no room for exception. Be on guard for answer choices that have definitive words such as *exactly* and *always.*

✓ Switchback Words

Stay alert for *switchbacks.* These are the words and phrases frequently used to alert you to shifts in thought. The most common switchback words are *but, although,* and *however.* Others include *nevertheless, on the other hand, even though, while, in spite of, despite,* and *regardless of.* Switchback words are important to catch because they can change the direction of the question or an answer choice.

☑ Face Value

When in doubt, use common sense. Accept the situation in the problem at face value. Don't read too much into it. These problems will not require you to make wild assumptions. If you have to go beyond creativity and warp time or space in order to have an answer choice fit the question, then you should move on and consider the other answer choices. These are normal problems rooted in reality. The applicable relationship or explanation may not be readily apparent, but it is there for you to figure out. Use your common sense to interpret anything that isn't clear.

Answer Choice Strategies

☑ Answer Selection

The most thorough way to pick an answer choice is to identify and eliminate wrong answers until only one is left, then confirm it is the correct answer. Sometimes an answer choice may immediately seem right, but be careful. The test writers will usually put more than one reasonable answer choice on each question, so take a second to read all of them and make sure that the other choices are not equally obvious. As long as you have time left, it is better to read every answer choice than to pick the first one that looks right without checking the others.

☑ Answer Choice Families

An answer choice family consists of two (in rare cases, three) answer choices that are very similar in construction and cannot all be true at the same time. If you see two answer choices that are direct opposites or parallels, one of them is usually the correct answer. For instance, if one answer choice says that quantity x increases and another either says that quantity x decreases (opposite) or says that quantity y increases (parallel), then those answer choices would fall into the same family. An answer choice that doesn't match the construction of the answer choice family is more likely to be incorrect. Most questions will not have answer choice families, but when they do appear, you should be prepared to recognize them.

☑ Eliminate Answers

Eliminate answer choices as soon as you realize they are wrong, but make sure you consider all possibilities. If you are eliminating answer choices and realize that the last one you are left with is also wrong, don't panic. Start over and consider each choice again. There may be something you missed the first time that you will realize on the second pass.

☑ Avoid Fact Traps

Don't be distracted by an answer choice that is factually true but doesn't answer the question. You are looking for the choice that answers the question. Stay focused on what the question is asking for so you don't accidentally pick an answer that is true but incorrect. Always go back to the question and make sure the answer choice you've selected actually answers the question and is not merely a true statement.

☑ Extreme Statements

In general, you should avoid answers that put forth extreme actions as standard practice or proclaim controversial ideas as established fact. An answer choice that states the "process should be used in certain situations, if..." is much more likely to be correct than one that states the "process should be discontinued completely." The first is a calm rational statement and doesn't even make a definitive, uncompromising stance, using a hedge word *if* to provide wiggle room, whereas the second choice is far more extreme.

✓ Benchmark

As you read through the answer choices and you come across one that seems to answer the question well, mentally select that answer choice. This is not your final answer, but it's the one that will help you evaluate the other answer choices. The one that you selected is your benchmark or standard for judging each of the other answer choices. Every other answer choice must be compared to your benchmark. That choice is correct until proven otherwise by another answer choice beating it. If you find a better answer, then that one becomes your new benchmark. Once you've decided that no other choice answers the question as well as your benchmark, you have your final answer.

✓ Predict the Answer

Before you even start looking at the answer choices, it is often best to try to predict the answer. When you come up with the answer on your own, it is easier to avoid distractions and traps because you will know exactly what to look for. The right answer choice is unlikely to be word-for-word what you came up with, but it should be a close match. Even if you are confident that you have the right answer, you should still take the time to read each option before moving on.

General Strategies

✓ Tough Questions

If you are stumped on a problem or it appears too hard or too difficult, don't waste time. Move on! Remember though, if you can quickly check for obviously incorrect answer choices, your chances of guessing correctly are greatly improved. Before you completely give up, at least try to knock out a couple of possible answers. Eliminate what you can and then guess at the remaining answer choices before moving on.

✓ Check Your Work

Since you will probably not know every term listed and the answer to every question, it is important that you get credit for the ones that you do know. Don't miss any questions through careless mistakes. If at all possible, try to take a second to look back over your answer selection and make sure you've selected the correct answer choice and haven't made a costly careless mistake (such as marking an answer choice that you didn't mean to mark). This quick double check should more than pay for itself in caught mistakes for the time it costs.

✓ Pace Yourself

It's easy to be overwhelmed when you're looking at a page full of questions; your mind is confused and full of random thoughts, and the clock is ticking down faster than you would like. Calm down and maintain the pace that you have set for yourself. Especially as you get down to the last few minutes of the test, don't let the small numbers on the clock make you panic. As long as you are on track by monitoring your pace, you are guaranteed to have time for each question.

✓ Don't Rush

It is very easy to make errors when you are in a hurry. Maintaining a fast pace in answering questions is pointless if it makes you miss questions that you would have gotten right otherwise. Test writers like to include distracting information and wrong answers that seem right. Taking a little extra time to avoid careless mistakes can make all the difference in your test score. Find a pace that allows you to be confident in the answers that you select.

☑ Keep Moving

Panicking will not help you pass the test, so do your best to stay calm and keep moving. Taking deep breaths and going through the answer elimination steps you practiced can help to break through a stress barrier and keep your pace.

Final Notes

The combination of a solid foundation of content knowledge and the confidence that comes from practicing your plan for applying that knowledge is the key to maximizing your performance on test day. As your foundation of content knowledge is built up and strengthened, you'll find that the strategies included in this chapter become more and more effective in helping you quickly sift through the distractions and traps of the test to isolate the correct answer.

Now that you're preparing to move forward into the test content chapters of this book, be sure to keep your goal in mind. As you read, think about how you will be able to apply this information on the test. If you've already seen sample questions for the test and you have an idea of the question format and style, try to come up with questions of your own that you can answer based on what you're reading. This will give you valuable practice applying your knowledge in the same ways you can expect to on test day.

Good luck and good studying!

Assessment and Data Collection

Medical History and Review of Systems

Elements of Patient History

In addition to the physical assessment and review of systems, a patient history should include the following elements:

- **Biographical information**: Name, age, gender, ethnicity, marital status, occupation/profession
- **Family history/relationships**: Information about genetic diseases, genogram, health status of family members, family members' causes of death and ages at death, support systems, family system, and communication patterns
- **Physical environment**: Living arrangements, type of housing, homeless status, and environmental hazards
- **Cultural environment**: Attitudes and beliefs about wellness, sickness, death, complementary therapies, language spoken in the home, and customs
- **Spiritual environment**: Religious and/or spiritual beliefs, religious practices, belief system
- **Lifestyle**: Sexual preferences (straight, gay, bisexual, etc.), sexual habits (masturbation, multiple partners, high-risk behaviors), personal habits (sleeping, eating, exercising), and substance abuse (alcohol, drugs, nicotine)
- **Social environment**: Friends, relationships, clubs, social media, sports participation
- **Disability**: Physical disabilities (hearing, vision, smell), mobility disorders and need for assistive devices (walkers, canes, wheelchairs) and mental disabilities (cognitive impairment, psychiatric/psychological disorders)

Special History-Taking Challenges

Special history-taking challenges exist when dealing with special populations. The following considerations should be taken:

- **Silent patient**: Be patient, sensitive, and alert for nonverbal clues.
- **Talkative patient**: Allow the patient to speak freely for a few minutes and then periodically summarize.
- **Anxious patient**: Be patient, provide reassurance, explain all procedures.
- **Patient with multiple complaints**: Ask the patient to help prioritize issues.
- **Hostile/angry patient**: Remain calm, respond as appropriate.
- **Intoxicated patient**: Avoid cornering, belittling, or challenging the patient or asking the patient to lower voice or stop swearing. Remain calm and treat the patient with respect.
- **Depressed, crying patient**: Assess the severity of depression, listen, and remain supportive and non-judgmental.
- **Patient with language barrier**: Use a translator, utilize hand gestures, show equipment before using and point to the part of the body where the equipment will be used.
- **Patient with visual impairment**: Announce presence, explain all procedures verbally, tell the patient before touching them.
- **Patient with hearing impairment**: Determine if the patient has a hearing aid and obtain it if possible. Speak slowly and clearly facing patient for hearing deficit. If the patient has complete hearing loss, use writing use hand gestures and demonstrations to communicate.

Previous/Current Therapies

The patient history should include information about previous and current therapies:

- **Medications**: Note any previous and current prescribed medications, including dosages, frequency, and duration as well as the reason for the drug.
- **Allergies**: Make note of any drug allergies or reactions, history of anaphylaxis, other allergies (dust, foods, latex, animals, plants, pollens).
- **Vitamins, minerals, and herbal preparations**: Be aware of types, dosages, frequency, and duration. If using herbal preparations or those not readily identified, determine where they were obtained as some from overseas may include substances banned in the US or dangerous to the health.
- **Complementary therapies**: Complementary therapies include relaxation, visualization, homeopathy, acupuncture, music therapy, aromatherapy, Ayurveda, biofeedback, chiropractic medicine, hypnosis, meditation, massage, traditional Chinese medicine, yoga, naturopathy, reflexology, acupuncture, and Tai Chi.
- **Cultural therapies**: Cultural therapies include the use of healers, shamans, coining, cupping, pricking (with a needle).
- **Fasting and cleanses**: Note the specific program, duration, and substances utilized for cleanses (oral, rectal).

Problem-Based Assessment for Chief Complaint

Patients often present with a myriad of health problems, so a **problem-based assessment**, focused on finding a solution to chief complaints and current health problems, can be effective. Problem-based assessment requires a thorough history to create a problem list. This approach does not preclude a complete exam, which might identify problems that the patient has neglected, but the focus remains on the problem list generated. The list should be prioritized to ensure that the most critical issues (blood in the stool) are thoroughly assessed before less critical issues (occasional insomnia). Once a problem is identified, then differential diagnoses are determined. With patients, especially adults, there may be a combination of physical and psychosocial elements to a problem. For example, urinary problems may relate to dehydration, lack of mobility, poor hygiene, medications, or disease. Appropriate diagnostic tests, further assessments, and interventions are completed as needed to diagnose and resolve problems.

Data Collection from Relevant Sources

During the initial assessment, the nurse **gathers information** about the patient's history. The interview should occur in a space that allows for some privacy but is not isolated in case the nurse needs assistance. Asking open-ended questions in a non-judgmental manner, "What problem brings you to the hospital?" is more effective than asking yes/no questions. Questions should focus on one problem or symptom at a time, for example, "How are your sleeping habits?" Depending on the patient's condition, information may be obtained by:

- Directly interviewing the patient
- Observing the patient's behavior and interactions with others
- Reviewing previous hospitalization and discharge records
- Carrying out diagnostic procedures (lab, imaging)

- Interviewing family or caregivers (If possible, some of the interview should be conducted outside of the patient's presence as people may speak more freely. However, the nurse must use care not to violate the patient's right to privacy and should, when possible, ask the patient for permission to speak to others.)
- Interviewing EMT or police and reviewing their written reports

Physical Examination

System-Based Physical Examination

A system-based physical examination is carried out methodically, moving from one system to another to ensure that all body systems are reviewed. The examination begins with a patient and family history and then a general survey that includes assessment of psychosocial status, substance abuse, domestic partner violence, measurements (height, weight), and vital signs as well as assessment of pain level and nutritional assessment. **System-based physical examination** utilizes inspection, palpation, percussion, and auscultation. While the order may vary somewhat, the usual order of examination is:

- Skin, nails, and hair
- Head, face, and neck
- Eyes, ears, nose, mouth, and throat
- Breasts and regional lymph nodes
- Thorax and lungs
- Heart and neck vessels
- Peripheral vascular/lymphatic system
- Abdomen
- Musculoskeletal system (may include functional assessment)
- Genitourinary system
- Anus, rectum, and prostate

Elements of Systems Review

General	Normal weight, changes in weight, sleeping patterns, malaise, weakness, and fever
Head	Frequency or occurrence of headaches, head injuries. Frequency of upper respiratory infections, nasal stuffiness, discharge, itching, hay fever, sinus congestion, and nosebleeds. Condition of teeth and gums, last dental exam, hoarseness, bleeding gums, sore tongue, and frequency of sore throats
Neck	Swollen lymph nodes, stiffness, and goiter
Eyes	Vision (contacts, glasses), redness, tearing, visual disturbances, glaucoma, cataracts, and macular degeneration
Ears	Hearing, vertigo, tinnitus, earaches, and discharge
Skin	Rashes, texture changes, jaundice, nevi, dryness, and lesions
Breasts	Masses, nipple discharge, changes in nipple, date of last mammogram, and frequency of SBE
Cardiac	Heart problems, hypertension, heart murmurs, chest pain, paroxysmal nocturnal dyspnea and prior ECGs or heart tests
Respiratory	Cough, sputum, dyspnea, hemoptysis, bronchitis, COPD, asthma, TB, pleurisy, and last chest x-ray and/or PPD
Gastrointestinal	Dysphagia, heartburn, appetite, nausea, vomiting, regurgitation, indigestions, frequency and character of stools, abdominal pain, food allergies/intolerances, flatus, jaundice, and hepatitis, liver, or gallbladder problems
Urinary	Frequency, nocturia, polyuria, pain or burning, hematuria, urgency, incontinence, changes in urinary stream, urinary infections, and calculi
Peripheral/Vascular	Leg pain, cramping, varicose veins, and phlebitis
Gynecological	Age at menarche/menopause, regularity, frequency, and duration of menses, bleeding between periods/after intercourse, discharge, premenstrual tension, postmenopausal symptoms, itching, masses, gravida/para/abortus, contraception, and sexual problems
Musculoskeletal	Pains, stiffness, arthritis, gout, backaches, inflammatory changes, and limitations in mobility
Neurologic	Fainting, seizures, blackouts, paresis/paralysis, change in sensation (numbness, tingling), tremors, and involuntary movement
Hematologic	Bruising, bleeding, anemia, and past transfusions/reactions
Endocrine	Thyroid disease, heat/cold intolerance, diabetes, polyuria/polydipsia, excessive hunger, and excessive perspiration
Psychiatric	Mood/anxiety disorders, nervousness, tension, cognitive impairment

Assessment of Functional Abilities

ADL and IADL

Functional impairment may affect the ability to prepare and receive adequate fluids and nutrition. Functional assessment may include:

- **Activities of daily living (ADL)**: This assesses the ability to care for oneself, including dressing, bathing, and preparing food. Inability to carry out ADL may relate to physical impairment (paralysis, paresis, frailty), or cognitive impairment (dementia, confusion).

- **Instrumental activities of daily living (IADL)**: This assesses managing affairs (including finances), arranging transportation, using prosthetic devices, shopping, and telephoning. Inability to carry out IADL may relate to cognitive impairment, poverty, or inaccessibility and can prevent people from shopping for or ordering food.

Gait Speed, TUG, and POMA

Gait assessments include:

- **Gait speed** in 5 meters with slow gait (<0.6 m/second) predictive of limitations.
- **Timed up and go (TUG)**: Patient stands from chair with armrests, walks 3 meters, turns, and sits back down. Those requiring ≥14 seconds are at risk for falls (Normal: 7-10 seconds).
- **Performance-oriented mobility assessment (POMA)** tests mobility and gait under different conditions.

Index of Independence of Activities of Daily Living and Palliative Performance Scale

The **Index of Independence of Activities of Daily Living (Katz Index)** tool is a check list that does not use scores but rather evaluates the individual in 6 areas (bathing, dressing, toileting, transfer, continence, and feeding) to provide an assessment of the person's need for assistance and progression of disease and/or disability.

The **Palliative Performance Scale** assesses the functional ability of older adults receiving palliative care. Categories are assessed by percentage of ability from 0% (death) to 100% with lower percentages indicative of functional impairment. The scores are used as a guide to determine probable life expectancy with 60-100% at 108 days, 30-50% at 41 days, and 10-20% at 6 days although survival rates have been primarily correlated with cancer rather than other terminal illness. Categories include:

- Ability to ambulate
- Activity level and evidence of disease
- Self-care
- Intake
- Level of consciousness

Assessing the Quality of Life

QOLS

The Quality-of-Life Scale (QOLS) is a self-administered test often used with adults, including the chronically ill, to assess the patient's perception of their quality of life. The tool has 7 categories with a total of 16 elements that are assessed with a 1-7 scale that ranges from satisfaction to dissatisfaction. The possible scores range from 16-112 with an average normal finding of about 90. The higher the score, the higher the perceived quality of life. Categories include:

- **Material/physical wellbeing**: Includes material wellbeing/financial security as well as health and personal safety
- **Interpersonal relationships**: Includes family members, spouse, children, and friends
- **Activities (social, community, civic)**: Includes those activities that involve assisting others and those related to local/national government
- **Personal development/fulfillment**: Includes intellectual development, personal understanding, creative expression, and role in occupation

- **Recreation**: Hobbies and leisure activities
- **Independence**: The ability to live and manage independently

Environmental Considerations

Environmental factors should be assessed within the actual environment if at all possible. If not, careful questioning and drawing of diagrams and approximate floor plans with the patient—or asking the patient to do drawings—can be useful, especially when showing the patient needed modifications. Family members may also assist with the assessment, providing useful information. Some patients, especially the elderly, may be reluctant to admit that the home is cluttered or that they are unable to maintain the home environment in a sanitary condition. Brochures and handouts about home safety and assistive devices should be provided to the patient as well as contact names and telephone numbers for equipment needed in the home. A checklist should be compiled of all necessary changes or additions, with specific details, such as "Install 18-inch grab bar across from toilet." In some cases, a social worker or occupational therapist should visit the patient.

Environmental Adaptations

Adaptations needed in the environment may vary widely for the hospice or palliative care patient:

- **Access issues**: If the patient needs to use a wheelchair, furniture may need to be moved, doorways widened, and wheelchair ramp installed. If the bathroom is difficult to access (upstairs, not wheelchair accessible), a bedside commode may be needed. Items may need to be moved or placed so they are easier to reach.
- **Safety issues**: Grab bars may need to be installed in bathrooms, hallways, and stairways and scatter rugs removed. Lighting may need to be improved. Patients may need assistive devices, such as wheelchairs, canes, and walkers. If patients are confused/disoriented/wandering, the home may need door latches, movement alarms, and other safety devices.
- **Equipment issues**: The patient may need a hospital bed or other equipment to facilitate care or relieve symptoms, and this can involve changes in wiring, moving furniture, and sometimes changing rooms.

Environmental Risk Factors

When assessing a patient, it is important to consider that certain environmental factors may place the patient at increased risk or may be a factor in disease. There are a number of different types of environmental factors:

Factors	Examples	Effects
Toxic chemicals	Lead, arsenic, muriatic acid, sulfuric acid, ammonia, lime	May result in poisoning (lead, arsenic) or burns (acids, ammonia, lime)
Physical objects	Guns, cars, knives, equipment	Accidents, gunshot wounds, stabbings, various injuries
Biological organisms	Bacteria, fungi, viruses	Infections
Temperature variations	Heat, cold	Burns, dehydration, heat stroke, hypothermia, frostbite
Ambient noise	Sirens, loud music, traffic noise, work-related noise	Hearing loss/deafness
Psychosocial	Increased stress	Anxiety, hypertension

Environmental Assessment

Environmental assessments are very helpful when developing a care plan to provide for care and safety. **Rooms should be assessed** according to their function:

- Entryway should be free of obstacles and surfaces even. Handrails and/or ramps may be needed for those who are unsteady or wheelchair bound.
- Stairs/steps should have handrails, non-skid surfaces, and contrast markings for each step.
- Living area should be comfortable and furniture arranged for convenience. Chairs should be firm enough for people to stand from easily.
- Bedrooms should have a night light and phone near the bed. Bed should be positioned close to the nearest bathroom if possible and at the appropriate height for easy access and appropriate firmness.
- Bathrooms may require grab bars, hand-held shower, and elevated toilet seat, tub seat.
- Kitchen may need items moved for convenient access as well as a sturdy step stool. Unsafe equipment/tools should be removed.

Additional Environmental Considerations to Assess

Some elements of environmental assessment are not specific to rooms in the house but are general needs that must be met in order for people, especially the elderly or disabled, to remain safe:

- Environmental hazards such as piles of papers or trash on the floors, loose carpet or rugs, and cluttered pathways can cause falls and must be cleared, organized, or repaired.
- Lighting should be adequate enough for reading in all rooms and stairways.
- Heat and air conditioning must be adequate. The young and the elderly are especially susceptible to heat and cold injury.
- Sanitation should ensure that health hazards do not exist, such as from rotting food or infestations of cockroaches or rodents.
- Animals should be cared for adequately with access to food, water, toileting, and routine veterinary care.
- Smoke/chemicals in the environment may pose a hazard, such as exposure to cigarette smoking or cleaning materials.

Nutritional Assessment

Nutritional assessment should be done within the first 24 hours of care for hospitalized patients and at the first visit for others to ensure that nutritional requirements are met. The history and physical exam should include the following information about the previous 3 months:

- Changes in food intake, including number of meals eaten daily
- Weight loss (or gain)
- Episodes of depression or stress that may relate to dietary intake

A sample of a usual daily menu should be developed. Additional **screening** should include:

- Daily number of protein, fruit, grain, and vegetable servings
- Usual fluid intake, including type, amount, and frequency
- Method of feeding, independent or assisted
- Mobility
- Mental status
- Body mass index (BMI), mid-arm circumference, and calf circumference
- Living status (independent or dependent)
- Prescription and non-prescription drugs
- Pressure sores or other wounds or skin problems

Physical Assessment for Nutritional Deficiency

The physical assessment is an important part of nutritional assessment to determine malnutrition or problems with self-feeding:

- Hair may be dry and brittle or thinning.
- Skin may show poor turgor, ecchymosis, tears, pressure areas, ulcerations, abrasions, or other compromises.
- Mouth may show dry mucous membranes. Lips may have cheilosis, cracking at the corners, and scaly lips (riboflavin deficiency). Gums may be swollen or bleeding, teeth loose or needing care, or poorly fitting dentures. Tongue may be inflamed, dry, cracked, or have sores.
- Nails may become brittle. Spoon shaped or pale nail bed indicates low iron.
- Hands may be crippled or arthritic, making eating difficult.
- Vision may be compromised so that people can't see to prepare food or have difficulty feeding themselves.
- Mental status may be impaired to the point that people can't understand diet instructions or prepare or eat meals.
- Motor skills may decrease, including hand-mouth coordination or ability to hold utensils.

Psychosocial and Spiritual Assessment

Psychosocial Assessment

A psychosocial assessment should provide additional information to the physical assessment to guide the patient's plan of care and should include:

- **Previous hospitalizations and experience with healthcare**
- **Psychiatric history**: suicidal ideation, psychiatric disorders, family psychiatric history, history of violence and/or self-mutilation
- **Chief complaint**: patient's perception
- **Complementary therapies**: acupuncture, visualization, and meditation
- **Occupational and educational background**: employment, retirement, and special skills.
- **Social patterns**: family and friends, living situation, typical activities, support system.
- **Sexual patterns**: orientation, problems, and sex practices
- **Interests/abilities**: hobbies and sports
- **Current or past substance abuse**: type, frequency, drinking pattern, use of recreational drugs, and overuse of prescription drugs
- **Ability to cope**: stress reduction techniques
- **Physical, sexual, emotional, and financial abuse**: whether the individual feels safe at home or where they live
- **Spiritual/cultural assessment**: religious/spiritual importance, practices, restrictions (such as blood products or foods), and impact on health/health decisions

Assessment of Patient/Family Knowledge of and Response to Advanced Illness

Assessment of patient/family knowledge of and response to advanced illness begins with a determination of how much they actually know about the illness and how much they want to know through direct interview and questioning. This includes questions like, "What do you understand about your disease?" and "What do you want to know about your disease?" Open-ended questions (as opposed to those answered with "yes" or "no") are most effective in eliciting information. Questioning can help evaluate the patient's/family's general health literacy and cognitive abilities as well as readiness to learn (related to physical, emotional, experiential, and knowledge readiness). Issues that should be covered during the **assessment include patient/family understanding** of:

- Disease and disease process
- Medications or treatments
- Adverse effects
- Signs and symptoms, including progression over time
- Prognosis
- End-of-life options for care
- Personal preferences

During the assessment, it's important to note both the patient's verbal and nonverbal communication and to remain supportive and non-judgmental.

Assessment of Patient/Family Support Systems

Patient/family **support systems** may vary widely and can include those that provide physical and/or emotional support:

- **Family members**: Family members (parents, spouse, siblings, children, grandparents) remain the primary support system for many patients and family, especially if they live nearby and can provide assistance, though even distant communication can provide emotional support.
- **Friends**: Close friends may provide support in lieu or in addition to family members and may, in some cases, be more aware of emotional needs because of longstanding close association.
- **Co-workers**: Co-workers may donate sick time, ease workload, and provide support in various manners.
- **Organizations**: Community organizations may help in provision of meals, transportation, visitors, and other types of support.
- **Religion/Spirituality**: Some religions/spiritual organizations provide not only emotional support but also nursing care and financial assistance.
- **Online support groups/message boards**: Internet support systems, such as message boards for specific types of cancer, can provide emotional support as well as useful information on treatment and coping.

Spiritual Assessments

HOPE Mnemonic

HOPE is a simple mnemonic used as a guideline for the spiritual assessment:

H	Hope	What sources of hope (who or what) do you have to turn to?
O	Organized	Are you a part of an organized religion or faith group? What do you gain from membership in this group?
P	Personal	What spiritual practices (prayer, meditation) are most helpful?
E	Effects	What effects do your beliefs play on any medical care or end-of-life issues and decisions? Do you have any beliefs that may affect the type of care the health care team can provide you with?

FICA Mnemonic

FICA is another abbreviated spiritual assessment tool:

F	Faith	Do you have a faith or belief system that gives your life meaning?
I	Importance	What importance does your faith have in your daily life?
C	Community	Do you participate and gain support from a faith community?
A	Address	What faith issues would you like me to address in your care?

SPIRIT Mnemonic

SPIRIT (Maugens) is a mnemonic used for a spiritual assessment tool:

S	Spiritual	Do you have a formal religious affiliation?
P	Personal	Which practices and beliefs do you personally accept and practice? Does spirituality play a part in your daily life?
I	Integration	Do you participate in a spiritual community and receive support from that community?

R	Ritual	Are there specific practices and restrictions in your religious convictions that would affect your healthcare choices?
I	Implication	Are there aspects of your spirituality you would like me to keep in mind during your care?
T	Terminal events	As you prepare for the end of life, how does your faith affect the decisions you make or how you feel about death?

SPIRITUAL CARE AT THE END OF LIFE

The patient's basic beliefs should be assessed in order to provide holistic care as the end of life approaches. **Spiritual care** must be provided according to the patient's religion and/or philosophy of choice, and must remain unbiased from the caregiver's own beliefs. If the patient does not wish to have spiritual counseling, it should not be pressed upon them. Advice and comfort can be provided by anyone known to the patient. Spiritual care is intended to relieve spiritual suffering and to explore answers to significant questions that the patient and family may have. Even those who do not have a formal religion affiliation or philosophical practice may experience questions and may search for meaning and comfort at the end of life.

The caregiver must assess prior and present religious affiliations, along with individual beliefs about God and the afterlife. The information must include devotional practices, rituals, and routines, and identify the degree of involvement and support available from the patient's chosen religious community. This spiritual assessment opens the door for effective spiritual caregiving, and it allows patients and their families to access spiritual coping strategies and support mechanisms. The holistic assessment addresses the patient's ability to resolve meaningful spiritual questions, identifying deeper understandings and retaining hope, strength, and peace. Questions can include the patient's interpretation of the meaning and purpose of their life, the role of family, and personal strengths and connections to various spiritual communities and to nature. Provisions should be made to explore spiritual relationships and to provide support for loss and crisis, as desired by the patient and family.

ADDRESSING EMOTIONAL AND SPIRITUAL HEALTH

Strategies to address emotional and spiritual health include:

- Remain observant and note both verbal and nonverbal communication.
- Address the patient by the surname unless asked to do otherwise, avoiding terms such as "honey" and "dear."
- Take the time to converse with the patient before broaching serious subjects.
- Use a pleasant and soft tone of voice when talking with the patient.
- Note indications of spiritual beliefs, such as Bibles, Korans, offering bowls, prayer beads, rosaries, and religious symbols as well as prayers, meditation, chants, signs of the cross, and fasts.
- Ask the meaning of unfamiliar symbols or items.
- Respect personal space, including noting how close the patient and family members stand to others.
- Avoid judgmental statements or attitudes toward traditions and practices that are different from those common to Western culture.
- Assist with religious or spiritual rituals and practices if requested.
- Ask the patient and family members if their needs are being met and about what issues are important to them.

Advanced Care Planning

Developing Plan of Care

The patient's plan of care is based on different types of **goals**:

- **Patient/family goals for care and outcomes** are a primary concern, especially for hospice and palliative care patients, whose care focuses on comfort and emotional support. These goals may relate to goals of life closure. Families, including young children, often want to be involved in developing the plan of care because participation increases feelings of self-worth and respect for healthcare providers.
- **Clinical needs/obligations** are aimed at preventing complications, treating disorders, and promoting comfort. The plan should focus on the problem list identified as part of the history and physical examination. Each item in the problem list must be addressed in the plan of care, including interventions, nursing goals (immediate, intermediate, and long-term), and expected outcomes and utilization of appropriate clinical pathways that are realistic for the patient's condition.

Review Video: Plan of Care
Visit mometrix.com/academy and enter code: 300570

Prioritizing Nursing Diagnoses and Problems

One method of prioritizing nursing and/or differential diagnoses is to consider consequences (high, medium, low) if treatment is delayed:

- **High** (Life threatening): Acute myocardial infarction, suicidal ideation
- **Medium** (Delay may cause problems): Malnutrition, manic episodes
- **Low** (Treatment can be delayed safely): Osteoarthritis, mild anxiety

Needs can also be prioritized according to **Maslow's Hierarchy of Needs**. American psychologist Abraham Maslow defined human motivation in terms of needs and wants. His hierarchy of needs is classically portrayed as a pyramid sitting on its base divided into horizontal layers. He theorized that, as humans fulfill the needs of one layer, their motivation turns to the layer above.

Self-actualization
desire to become the most that one can be
Esteem
respect, self-esteem, status, recognition, strength, freedom
Love / Belonging
friendship, intimacy, family, sense of connection
Safety needs
personal security, employment, resources, health, property
Physiological needs
air, water, food, shelter, sleep, clothing, reproduction

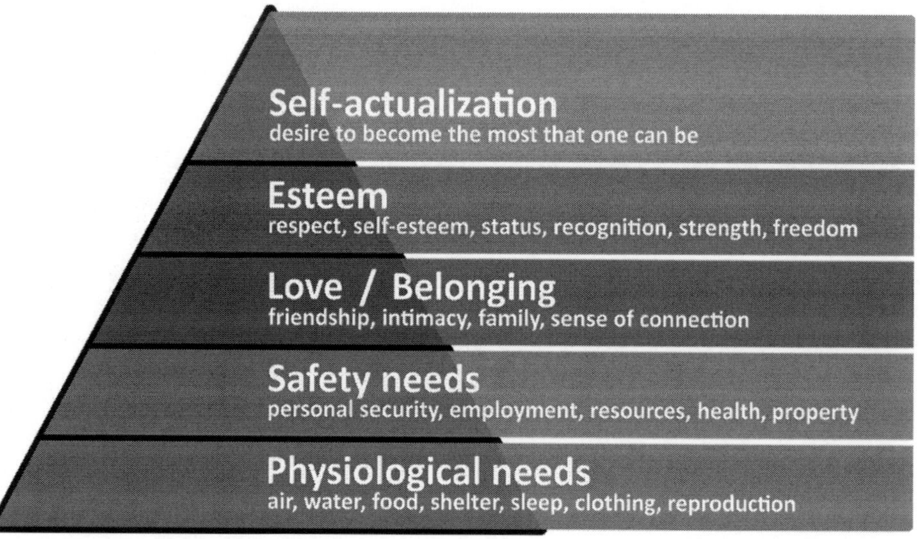

Level	Need	Description
Physiological	Basic needs to sustain life—oxygen, food, fluids, sleep	These basic needs take precedence over all other needs and must be dealt with first before individuals can focus on other needs.
Safety and security	Freedom from physiological and psychological threats	Once basic needs are met, individuals become concerned about safety, including freedom from fear, job security, war, and disasters. Children respond more intensely to threats than adults.
Love/Belonging	Support, caring, intimacy	Individuals tend to avoid isolation and loneliness and have a need for family, intimacy, or membership in a group where they feel they belong.
Self-esteem	Sense of worth, respect, independence	To have confidence, individuals need to develop self-esteem and receive the respect of others.
Self-actualization	Meeting one's own sense of potential and finding fulfillment	Individuals choose a path in life that leads to fulfillment and contentment.

Review Video: Maslow's Hierarchy of Needs
Visit mometrix.com/academy and enter code: 461825

Assisting Patient/Family in Evaluating Resources

The steps in assisting patient/family in evaluating appropriate and available resources includes:

- Develop a problem list and plan of care in collaboration with patient and family.
- Identify needs associated with plan of care, including those associated with hospitalization and home care.
- Categorize needs as follows:
    - **General care**: Hospital bed, bedpan, wheelchair, walker, assistive devices, meal preparation (home, Meals-on-Wheels)
    - **Treatment**: Medications, dressings, IVs, catheters, nutritional supplements
    - **Transportation**: Availability and requirements (car, ambulance, bus, taxi)
    - **Financial**: Insurance/Medicare coverage, co-pay, income, savings
    - **Caregiver**: Who will provide care, how often, where, when, and how, including the need to hire caregivers; need for respite care and/or homemaking services
    - **Consultation/Therapy**: Speech therapy, physical therapy, occupational therapy, etc.
    - **Psychological care**: Counseling, support programs
- Review categories and determine where additional resources are needed to ensure needs are met and what the patient/family can afford or attend to without further assistance.
- Provide lists of resources and/or referrals for deficits where additional resources are needed.

Unique Needs of Special Population

Certain populations require special considerations when developing their plan of care:

- **Substance abusers**: May need referral for drug/alcohol rehabilitation or drug maintenance (such as methadone) program. May require referrals for dental care and treatment of infections. Interventions may include dealing with drug-seeking behaviors and ongoing substance abuse.
- **Homeless**: May need treatment for lice and malnutrition. May need referral for psychiatric care and/or substance abuse (as above). Discharge planning may require assistance from social services and housing authorities.
- **Cognitively impaired**: Special interventions may be needed for safety, such as movement alarms, keeping side rails down, or attendants. Interventions may include alternative communication devices/approaches and dysphagia precautions. Consultation may be needed regarding effective management.
- **Elderly**: Fall and dysphagia precautions are often needed as well as functional assessment to ensure the patient receives adequate assistance with ADLS. This population may need nutritional supplementation and monitoring of intake and output and bowel movements.
- **Veterans**: Any of the needs/interventions above may apply. Interventions to deal with PTSD include determining triggers and maintaining a quiet environment when possible.

Patient Goals/Outcomes

The plan of care is developed from information gained from patient interviews, history and physical exam, and medical records. Once a problem list is generated, the nurse must review and prioritize the list and determine **patient goals/outcomes**, depending on the type of problem. Goals should be specifically related to the problem, measurable by some method, and attainable:

- Some problems (such as cardiac arrhythmias) can improve with treatment, so goals will aim toward resolution: "Pulse rate will not exceed 90 at rest."
- Other problems (such as chronic conditions) probably won't resolve, so the goals will aim toward preventing deterioration or further complications: "Patient will maintain current weight."
- Some problems (terminal cancer) cannot be resolved and deterioration of condition is inevitable, so the goal will aim toward palliation and ensuring the patient's comfort and support: "Patient will not experience breakthrough pain."

Disease Progression and Prognostication

Autoimmune Disorders

HIV/AIDS

HIV (human immunodeficiency virus) is the retrovirus that causes AIDS (acquired immune deficiency syndrome). Diagnosis is determined by the CD4+ T-cell count with AIDS currently diagnosed with a CD4+ count of <200 cells per mm^3. HIV is transmitted in bodily fluids (blood, semen, vaginal secretions, breast milk) that contain free virions and infected CD4+ T-cells. Categories of HIV include:

- **Category A**: (CD4+ count <500). Asymptomatic or lymphadenopathy, sore throat, fatigue.
- **Category B**: (CD4+ count 200-499). Conditions include candidiasis, pelvic inflammatory disease, bacillary angiomatosis, fever, diarrhea, herpes zoster, low platelet count, weight loss, and peripheral neuropathy.
- **Category C (AIDS)**: (CD4+ count <200). Late-stage illness. Invasive diseases are common.

Risk factors include unprotected sex, especially males having sex with other males, and needle sharing. Patients often need support in dealing with anxiety, coping with increasing symptoms, adhering to medical protocols, and finding meaning and value in their lives.

Effects on Cells

The **AIDS virus** attaches itself to the **CD4 cell surface protein** of T-4 lymphocytes with a viral envelope of glycoprotein (gp120). This protein binds to CD4 receptors and coreceptors (CXCR4 and CCR5). HIV is a **retrovirus** that quickly infects circulating immune cells or finds safe harbors in body reservoirs that are inaccessible to drug therapy. The retrovirus uses an enzyme called **reverse transcriptase** to convert the HIV viral RNA to a viral DNA. This conversion allows the viral DNA to take over the host cell DNA of lymphocytes, macrophages, and other immune system cells. When the viral DNA has taken over, it produces viral proteins that assemble into **virions** using viral enzyme protease. Each reproductive cycle of HIV can produce up to 100 billion virions with minor protective mutations.

Common Associated Infections and Malignancies

The AIDS patient is highly **susceptible** to many bacterial, viral, fungal, and parasitic infections as well as certain types of cancers, such as Kaposi sarcoma, Hodgkin's lymphoma, and non-Hodgkin's lymphoma.

- **Bacterial infections** include *Streptococcus pneumoniae, Mycobacterium intracellulare* (MAI) and Mycobacterium avium complex (MAC), tuberculosis (TB), salmonellosis, syphilis, and Bacillary angiomatosis.
- **Viral infections** include cytomegalovirus (CMV), viral hepatitis, herpes simplex virus (HSV), human papillomavirus (HPV), and progressive multifocal leukoencephalopathy (PML).
- **Fungal infections** include Candida albicans, Histoplasma capsulatum, and cryptococcal meningitis.
- **Parasitic infections** include toxoplasmosis and cryptosporidium.

The rates of infection with these types of infections in AIDS patients far exceed the rates found within the general population.

AIDS Dementia Complex

The exact cause of **AIDS dementia** is unknown, but it is a primary result of the disease process of AIDS itself. Current theories suggest that the HIV infection stimulates an invasion of **macrophages** in the brain (microglia). These release **cytokines** that directly damage the nervous tissue by disrupting the neurotransmitter functions and cause encephalopathy. This condition affects as many as 15% of all AIDS patients. Prognosis is poor, and the disease is not reversible. However, **retrovirals** can delay its onset. Central nervous system HIV infection in children tends to have a more dramatic and pronounced effect than that in adults. AIDS dementia is characterized by gradual memory loss, decreased concentration, and cognition and mood disorders. The patient may also experience physical symptoms of ataxia, incontinence, and seizures.

Systemic Lupus Erythematosus

Systemic lupus erythematosus is a systemic reaction to collagen or connective tissue in the body, believed to be triggered by an antibody-antigen immune response to an environmental agent, resulting in widespread damage of vessels and organs, primarily in females. Onset is usually age 9-15 and is more common in African American, Hispanic, and Asian females than Caucasian.

Symptoms (vary widely)	Treatment (varies with severity)
• Butterfly rash (scaly erythematous maculopapular patches) on face, chest, and arms. • Arthritic-type pain, stiffness, and swelling of joints. • CNS involvement with seizures, headache, and psychosis. • Heart/vessels (pericarditis, vasculitis) and lung (pleurisy) inflammation. • Kidney failure. • Anemia (erythrocytopenia and pancytopenia, hemolytic). • Spleen, liver, and lymph nodes enlarged. • GI symptoms: Nausea, vomiting, pain, and hepatitis.	• NSAIDs for pain and inflammation. • Steroids for organ inflammation and hemolytic anemia. • Antimalarial drugs for skin involvement. • Immunosuppressant agents if steroids not adequate. • Patients may need support dealing with fatigue (rest, energy-conservation methods), pain, decreased mobility, nutrition, and anxiety/depression.

Rheumatoid Arthritis

Rheumatoid arthritis is a chronic systemic autoimmune inflammatory disorder of the connective tissue of synovial joints, resulting in loss of cartilage and joint deformity. RA has onset at 25 to 50 years, usually beginning with pain and stiffness in the hands, wrists, and feet. Joint inflammation and deformity increases over time. Symptoms include pain, stiffness, swelling, erythema, nodules, and lack of function in affected joints, and generalized weakness, fatigue, weight loss, and fever. Involvement is systemic, bilateral, and symmetric. Treatment includes light exercise to prevent contractures and pharmacologic treatment: salicylates (ASA), NSAIDs, COX-2 inhibitors (Celebrex), disease-modifying antirheumatic drugs (gold-containing compounds, methotrexate, azathioprine, adalimumab), immunomodulator (abatacept), interleukin-1 receptor inhibitors (anakinra), and glucocorticoids (prednisone) and topical analgesics. RA may be classified according to joint damage and/or functional status. Those in class 4 (functional) generally have limitations in ability to carry out all activities and require assistance in all ADLs. Patients often experience severe fatigue because of joint pain and disturbed sleep, so patients may especially need support in managing pain and conserving energy.

Oncologic Disorders

End-Stage Disease Progression of Oncologic Disorders

End-stage progression of oncologic disorders may vary depending on the type of cancer and the areas of metastasis but often includes the following:

- **Pain**: This is the most common complication and may be localized or generalized. Opioids are the treatment of choice, usually on a continuous round-the-clock schedule with additional doses for breakthrough pain at end-stage to provide as much comfort as possible.
- **Nausea/vomiting**: Anti-emetics and/or medical marijuana may help to reduce nausea and vomiting. The patient's diet should be altered to include those foods the patient can best tolerate, often soft, bland, or liquid foods.
- **Dyspnea**: Dyspnea is common, and supplementary oxygen may help to provide some relief.
- **Confusion**: Supportive care and reorienting the patient may help to reduce confusion, but confusion often persists, especially with high doses of opioids.
- **Bowel/bladder dysfunction**: This is common because of dehydration and opioid use. Stool softeners, laxatives and encouraging fluid intake may help. If the patient is still able to eat, adding yogurt, fiber, and prune juice to the diet may be helpful.

Advanced Renal Cancer

Renal cancers generally occur **asymptomatically** in the early stages. Symptoms begin to appear as the condition worsens. Gross hematuria, dull, aching pain, and palpable abdominal mass are generally the first signs. When all three of these are evidenced in the patient, it is generally a well-advanced cancer. **Hematuria** is the most common symptom but may not be noticed until it has reached the gross stage where it is visible to the naked eye. Other late signs and symptoms can include fever, anemia, weight loss, night sweats, elevated erythrocyte sedimentation rate, dyspnea, hypertension, hypercalcemia, and polycythemia. **Polycythemia** may cause headaches, dizziness, vein inflammation, itchiness, and a general feeling of bloating. **Hypercalcemia** causes tiredness, decreased appetite, frequent urination, thirst, nausea, vomiting, confusion, difficulty concentrating, and constipation.

Renal Failure

When the kidneys become unable to function, either short or long-term, it is referred to as renal failure. Causes for kidney failure range from toxins (including some medications that may become nephrotoxic), tumors, infections, diabetes, and hypertension to collagen vascular diseases such as lupus. When there is hope of restoring normal kidney function, peritoneal dialysis or hemodialysis as well as diuretics and the treatment of underlying causes such as hypertension may be used. Dietary treatments typically focus on a low sodium, low protein, and low potassium regimen. Dialysis, and its supplementary treatments, is the treatment of choice for chronic kidney failure. When there is no hope of return to normal kidney function, the patient faces the difficult decision of whether or not to start, continue, or even stop dialysis. This decision will either prolong the patient's life or bring death within just a few days. As the disease progresses it brings more pronounced complications in fluid and electrolyte balances, anemia, and uremia. At this point, the patient's treatment may turn to a focus on comfort and palliative medications rather than on prolonging life by the use of dialysis.

Leukemia

Leukemia is an acute or chronic condition in which proliferating white blood cells compete with normal cells for nutrition. Leukemia affects all cells because the abnormal cells in the bone marrow depress the formation of all elements, resulting in the following consequences, regardless of the type of leukemia:

- Decrease in production of erythrocytes (RBCs), resulting in anemia.
- Decrease in neutrophils, resulting in increased risk of infection.
- Decrease in platelets, with subsequent decrease in clotting factors and increased bleeding or hemorrhage with pallor petechiae, purpura, and bleeding mucous membranes. Patients may need guidance regarding dental care.
- Increased risk of physiological fractures because of invasion of bone marrow that weakens the periosteum.
- Infiltration of liver, spleen, and lymph glands, resulting in enlargement and fibrosis.
- Infiltration of the CNS, resulting in increased intracranial pressure, ventricular dilation, and meningeal irritation with headaches, vomiting, papilledema, nuchal rigidity, and coma progressing to death.
- Hypermetabolism that deprives cells of nutrients, resulting in anorexia, weight loss, muscle atrophy, and fatigue. Patients often need support regarding nutrition and fatigue.

Colorectal Cancers

Colorectal cancers are the third most common cancer, and adenocarcinomas account for up to 95% of all colorectal cancers. There are two additional subtypes of adenocarcinomas that are less common:

- **Signet ring** is a very aggressive form that is harder to treat but accounts for only 0.1% of adenocarcinomas.
- **Mucinous** is also an aggressive form that is composed of about 60% mucous, allowing the cells to spread faster and making it hard to treat. This form accounts for 10-15% of adenocarcinomas.

Because symptoms often do not appear before the disease is advanced, many patients will undergo colectomy with re-anastomosis or with formation of a colostomy, which requires ongoing care. Patients with advanced disease may be unable to care for a colostomy independently, and the psychological impact of the stoma may be profound. Patients need not only physical support for pain and colostomy care but also often emotional support to deal with changing body image and depression.

Lung Cancer

Lung cancer is the most common cause of cancer-related deaths. Symptoms vary with type of tumor but are often not evident until metastasis has occurred. The most common symptom is cough that changes in character. Later symptoms include hemoptysis, dyspnea, weight loss, fatigue, nausea and vomiting, hoarseness, dysphagia, and unilateral diaphragmatic paralysis. Lung cancers may be primary, arising within the tissue of the lung, or secondary, spreading from a distant tumor. Secondary tumors can be identified by the type of tumor cells, as the cells are the same as those of the primary tumor site. Most primary lung cancers arise from the lining of the bronchi or bronchioles. Treatment may include surgical excision, radiotherapy, and/or chemotherapy, depending on the type and stage of the tumor. Most forms of lung cancer are associated with cigarette smoking or exposure to second-hand smoke. Even after treatment, dyspnea is common, and the nurse must be alert for signs of metastasis (most commonly to adrenals, bone, brain, liver, or other lung sites).

Breast Cancer

The most common type (75%) of breast cancer is infiltrating ductal carcinoma. This cancer progresses from ductal carcinoma in situ and originates in ductal cells but spreads to adjacent tissue and often metastasizes to axillary nodes. Treatment includes lumpectomy with radiation or mastectomy. If lymph nodes are positive, chemotherapy may be administered. Follow-up treatment depends on whether the cancer is hormone receptive and may include trastuzumab (Herceptin), tamoxifen, or aromatase inhibitor (Femara). Patients must deal with pain, fear of metastasis (most commonly to bone, brain, liver, or lung), and altered self-image, especially after mastectomy. About 15% develop cancer in the other breast. The nurse must be aware of the psychological impact of the disease and provide relief of symptoms but also encourage the patient to express feelings and help the patient to develop coping strategies. Anxiety and depression are common. Patients may benefit from peer support groups.

Prostate Cancer

Cancer of the prostate primarily occurs in older adults, average age 72. Many tumors are non-lethal or progress so slowly that they pose little threat to the person, but increased screening with PSA, ultrasound, and digital rectal exam in asymptomatic males has resulted in earlier diagnosis and more aggressive treatment. Both benign prostatic hypertrophy and prostatic carcinoma are frequently treated with transurethral resection of the prostate (TURP), especially if the volume of the gland reaches only 40-50 mL. Prostate cancer tends to be more aggressive with earlier onset.

Signs and symptoms	Treatment
• Dysuria—difficulty initiating flow • Frequency, urgency • Hematuria • Bloody semen • Difficulty achieving erection • Lower back pain • Pain in hips and proximal thighs	Note: Treatment varies depending on age of onset, size of lesion, stage, and symptoms and may include one or more of the following: • Monitoring (watch and wait) • Surgical excision • Hormone therapy • Chemotherapy • Radiation • Supportive care to help the patient cope with pain, erectile dysfunction, impotence, and metastasis (most commonly to adrenals, bone, liver, and lungs)

Primary Hepatocellular Carcinoma

Primary hepatocellular carcinoma, the most common liver cancer, is usually associated with a history of cirrhosis (especially from chronic hepatitis) but can result from hemochromatosis or alcoholism. Even with removal, many cancers recur, especially if the tumor is >5 cm. Diagnostic findings include ultrasound, liver function tests, elevation of serum alpha fetoprotein (occurs in 70% in Western countries), elevation of serum des-gamma-carboxyl prothrombin (in 90%), abdominal CT, liver scan, and liver biopsy. Metastasis is commonly to the lungs and regional lymph nodes.

Signs and symptoms	Treatment
• Cachexia and loss of weight • Bruising • Fever • Splenomegaly • Hepatic bruit or friction rub • Lethargy • RUQ discomfort, sometimes radiating to right shoulder • Jaundice • Ascites (fluid may be bloody)	• Surgical removal or transplantation for small tumors <3 cm • Chemotherapy/radiation may shrink large masses prior to surgery, but response is usually poor. Transcatheter arterial chemoembolization (TACE) or chemoinfusion (TACI) into hepatic arteries may provide palliation. • Multikinase inhibitor (tumor blocking medication): Sorafenib (Nexavar) orally • Support care with analgesia (opioids)

Secondary Hepatic Cancer

Secondary hepatic cancer occurs more frequently than primary hepatic cancer because cancer cells in the blood filter through the liver from primary tumors throughout the body, such as pulmonary, colon, prostatic, gastric, renal, and breast cancers. Secondary hepatic cancer has characteristics of the primary tumor and may, in fact, be diagnosed first when symptoms indicate hepatic abnormality. Prognosis is poor because metastasis has already occurred. Diagnostic tests include ultrasound, liver function tests, and extreme drug resistance testing to determine the most effective chemotherapeutic agent, PET, and MRI. In some cases, liver biopsy may be needed, especially if the primary tumor has not been identified.

Signs and symptoms	Treatment
• Anorexia and loss of weight • Bruising • Fever • Splenomegaly • Lethargy • RUQ discomfort, sometimes radiating to right shoulder • Jaundice • Ascites	• Chemotherapy appropriate for the primary tumor may include TACE and/or TACI • Surgical removal/radiofrequency ablation of small lesions to reduce obstruction and spread • Cryosurgery • Supportive and/or palliative care, emotional support

Bladder Cancer

Bladder cancer and most other urinary cancers begin in the inside lining of the urinary organs (urothelium) and then invade the deeper layers.

Symptoms	Treatment
• **Gross hematuria**: Frank bright red blood may be evident. Sometimes urine is brown or rust-colored. This is usually the first sign of bladder cancer. Blood in urine may appear, disappear, and reappear, usually without pain. • **Microscopic hematuria**: Blood may be present but only visible under microscope examination. • **Dysuria**: Patient may have burning on urination or pain, the feeling that the bladder does not completely empty on urination, and frequency.	**Options include**: • Transurethral resection with fulguration • Radical or segmental cystectomy • Urinary diversion **Post-surgical options include**: • Chemotherapy • Radiation • Biologic therapy • Clinical trials • Supportive care

Brain Tumors

Brain tumors may be primary or secondary, resulting from metastasis from other organs. The most common primary neoplastic brain tumors in adults are astrocytoma and oligodendroglioma; and, in pediatric patients, medulloblastomas, astrocytoma, brain stem glioma, and ependymoma. Symptoms may vary widely but often include deficits in vision or hearing, ataxia, changes in mental status, nausea and vomiting, headaches, dizziness, paresthesias, and seizures. Diagnosis is usually through neurological exam and MRI. Treatment most often involves surgical excision of all or part of the tumor, radiotherapy, and/or chemotherapy. Patients may need to maintain head elevation after surgery to reduce cerebral edema and pressure, so they may need positioning assistance. Patients often need medications to control nausea and vomiting as well as pain. Some patients may exhibit personality changes (especially if the frontal lobe was involved), and family may need support in dealing with the changes.

Neurologic Disorders

Amyotrophic Lateral Sclerosis (ALS)

ALS is a rapidly progressing **degenerative neuromuscular disease** with an unknown origin. The main area of involvement is the **motor neurons** of the brain and spinal cord. Approximately half of those patients presenting with ALS will have difficulty swallowing as their first symptom. Other patients will experience distal weakness. As the disease progresses, weakness affects both the upper and lower neurons. Death generally results from **respiratory failure** due to weakness in the diaphragm along with decreased laryngeal and lingual functionality. Swallowing and oral nourishment are of high concern for these patients. Loss of motility in the tongue and hypopharynx result in the loss of ability to manipulate food as well as creating speech and communication barriers.

Review Video: Amyotrophic Lateral Sclerosis (ALS)
Visit mometrix.com/academy and enter code: 178603

Cerebrovascular Accidents

Cerebrovascular accidents most commonly occur in the right or left hemisphere, but the exact location and the extent of brain damage affects the type of presenting symptoms. If the frontal area of either side is involved, there tends to be memory and learning deficits. Some **symptoms** are common to specific areas and help to identify the area involved:

- **Right hemisphere**: This results in left paralysis or paresis and a left visual field deficit that may cause spatial and perceptual disturbances so that people may have difficulty judging distance. Fine motor skills may be impacted, resulting in trouble dressing or handling tools. People may become impulsive and exhibit poor judgment, often denying impairment. Left-sided neglect (lack of perception of things on the left side) may occur. Difficulty following directions, short-term memory loss, and depression are also common. Language skills usually remain intact.
- **Left hemisphere**: This results in right paralysis or paresis and a right visual field defect. Depression is common and people often exhibit slow, cautious behavior, requiring repeated instruction and reinforcement for simple tasks. Short-term memory loss and difficulty learning new material or understanding generalizations is common. Difficulty with mathematics, reading, writing, and reasoning may occur. Aphasia (expressive, receptive, or global) is common.
- **Brain stem**: Because the brain stem controls respiration and cardiac function, a brain attack (stroke) frequently causes death, but those who survive may have a number of problems, including respiratory and cardiac abnormalities. Strokes may involve motor or sensory impairment or both.
- **Cerebellum**: This area controls balance and coordination. Strokes in the cerebellum are rare but may result in ataxia, nausea and vomiting, and headaches and dizziness or vertigo.

Dementias

End-stage progression of **dementia** results in patients becoming increasingly confused and unable to care for themselves. They may eventually lose the ability to speak, walk, or carry out any ADLs and become bedridden and non-responsive. Patients with dementia are at increased **risk** for falls, dysphagia, pressure sores, aspiration, delirium, and seizures. Some patients may become aggressive or violent, especially if frightened or severely confused. In advanced stages, medications (such as cholinesterase inhibitors, which are used for mild to moderate dementia and NMDA antagonists, used to treat moderate to severe dementia) to **control behavior** or **improve cognition** may be of limited value. SSRIs, such as citalopram, sertraline, and duloxetine are sometimes used to treat associated depression or aggressive behavior when other strategies have been unsuccessful. Anticonvulsants, such as carbamazepine and sodium valproate, may help to control aggressive behavior, but antipsychotic drugs are generally avoided because of increased risk of death. The CHPN should maintain a calm, quiet environment and use a friendly tone of voice to speak to the patient, even if the patient cannot respond.

Alzheimer's Disease

In Alzheimer's disease, there is disruption in both the electrical activity and the neurotransmitters in the brain. The cerebral cortex begins to atrophy, especially in the area of the hippocampus, which controls storage of new memories, resulting in characteristic short-term memory loss. Seven stages of disease progression (Reisberg) include:

- **Stage 1**: Preclinical with no evident impairment
- **Stage 2**: Mild cognitive decline, misplaces items, forgets words
- **Stage 3**: Mild, early-stage, problems with reading, retention, planning, handling money, organizing
- **Stage 4**: Moderate cognitive decline, difficulty with complex tasks, social withdrawal, can manage most ADLs
- **Stage 5**: Moderately severe cognitive decline, obvious confusion and disorientation, difficulty using language and managing ADLs, dress inappropriately, forget to eat, forget address, telephone number
- **Stage 6**: Moderately severe cognitive decline, profoundly confused and unable to care for self, may wander, develop sundowner's syndrome and obsessive behavior
- **Stage 7**: Very severe, wheelchair/bedbound, lose ability to speak, incontinent, muscles weak and rigid, dysphagia occurs

Non-Alzheimer's Dementias

Dementia can result from various non-Alzheimer's related conditions, including the following:

- **Creutzfeldt-Jakob disease**: CJD causes rapidly progressive dementia with impaired memory, behavioral changes, and incoordination.
- **Dementia with Lewy Bodies**: Cognitive and physical decline is similar to Alzheimer's, but symptoms may fluctuate frequently. This form of dementia may include visual hallucinations, muscle rigidity, and tremors.
- **Fronto-temporal dementia**: This may cause marked changes in personality and behavior and is characterized by difficulty using and understanding language.
- **Mixed dementia**: Dementia mirrors Alzheimer's and another type because of two different causes of dementia.
- **Normal pressure hydrocephalus**: This is characterized by ataxia, memory loss, and urinary incontinence.
- **Parkinson's dementia**: This form of dementia may involve impaired decision making and difficulty concentrating, learning new material, understanding complex language, sequencing, inflexibility, and short or long-term memory loss.
- **Vascular dementia**: Memory loss may be less pronounced than that common to Alzheimer's, but symptoms are similar.

Cardiac Disorders

Heart Failure

Heart failure (HF) is a cardiac disease that includes disorders of contractions (systolic dysfunction) or filling (diastolic dysfunction) or both. It may include pulmonary, peripheral, or systemic edema. Congestive heart failure occurs in end-stage HF in which edema is pronounced. Left ventricular dysfunction usually precedes right. Common causes include coronary artery disease, systemic or pulmonary hypertension, cardiomyopathy, and valvular disorders. The incidence of chronic heart failure correlates with age. There are two main types of HF: systolic and diastolic. The **New York Heart Association classification** is based on function:

- **Class I**: The patient is essentially asymptomatic during normal activities with no pulmonary congestion or peripheral hypotension. There is no restriction on activities, and prognosis is good.
- **Class II**: Symptoms appear with physical exertion but are usually absent at rest, resulting in some limitations of ADL. Slight pulmonary edema may be evident by basilar rales. Prognosis is good.
- **Class III**: Obvious limitations of ADL and discomfort on any exertion. Prognosis is fair.
- **Class IV**: Symptoms at rest. Prognosis is poor.

Pericardial Effusion

Pericardial effusion is defined as an accumulation of fluid within the pericardial cavity. Effusions (whether pleural or pericardial) will affect nearly 20% of patients with lung cancer during the advanced stages of the disease. They are also associated with breast cancer, leukemia, and lymphoma. This condition carries a poor prognosis for these patients. Pericardial effusion can be caused by the presence of cancerous cells or by the treatments used in defense of these malignancies, as well as potentially having other nonmalignant causes. Other possible causes include pericarditis, congestive heart failure, uremia, myocardial infarction, autoimmune diseases, infections, hypothyroidism, and renal and hepatic failure. Clinical signs and symptoms are dependent on the amount of fluid, how quickly it accumulates, and the general health of the cardiac tissue. Dyspnea is the most common presenting symptom, and the patient may be unable to speak more than one word with each breath. There may also be complaints of chest heaviness, dry cough, and generalized weakness. Physically, tachycardia is present as the body tries to compensate for the reduced cardiac output.

Pulmonary Disorders

COPD

Functional dyspnea, body mass index (BMI), and spirometry are used to assess the stages of **COPD**. Spirometry measures used are the ratio of forced expiratory volume in the 1st second of expiration (FEV_1) after full inhalation to total forced vital capacity (FVC). Normal lung function decreases after age 35; so, normal values are adjusted for height, weight, gender, and age:

- **Stage I (mild)**: Minimal dyspnea with or without cough and sputum. FEV_1 is ≥80% of predicted rate and FEV_1: FVC <70%.
- **Stage 2 (moderate)**: Moderate to severe chronic exertional dyspnea with/without cough and sputum. FEV_1 is 50-80% of predicted rate and FEV_1: FVC <70%.
- **Stage 3 (severe)**: Same as stage 2 but repeated episodes with increased exertional dyspnea and condition impacting quality of life. FEV_1 is 30-50% of predicted rate and FEV_1: FVC <70%.
- **Stage 4 (very severe)**: Severe dyspnea and life-threatening episodes that severely impact quality of life. FEV_1 is 30% of predicted rate or <50% with chronic respiratory failure and FEV_1: FVC <70%.

Management of End-Stage COPD

End-stage COPD is characterized by severe dyspnea. Some patients may be confused from lack of oxygen, and tachycardia is common. **Management** includes:

- Bronchodilators, such as albuterol (Ventolin) and salmeterol (Serevent), may help relieve bronchospasm and airway obstruction.
- Corticosteroids, both inhaled (Pulmicort, Vanceril) and oral (prednisone) may improve symptoms but are used most for associated asthma. High doses may result in numerous adverse effects.
- Oxygen therapy may be long term continuous or used during exertion.
- Patients should be placed in a position of comfort, usually with the head elevated.
- Eating and drinking may exhaust patient, so small frequent feedings are best.
- Skin tears and bruising are common with steroid therapy, so patients must have frequent skin care and use appropriate pressure-reducing surfaces, especially for those who insist on sitting upright and move little.
- Remain patient and supportive because patients are often irritable because of poor oxygenation and general discomfort.

Pleural effusion

A pleural effusion occurs when fluid accumulates in the pleural space. Secretion rates are increased and/or fluid absorption becomes restricted causing excessive fluid to collect. The onset of a pleural effusion can be slow or rapid. The patient will most often present with dyspnea. Dyspnea generally results from the collapse of a lung due to increased pleural fluid pressure. The inability to expand the lung leads to the complaint of dyspnea. As the affected area increases, dyspneic distress also increases along with orthopnea and tachypnea, anorexia, malaise, and fatigue. The patient may also complain of a dry, nonproductive cough and an aching, heaviness, or dull pain in the chest. Treatment of a cancer-induced pleural effusion is palliative and symptomatic in nature, and is dependent on the surrounding circumstances, the overall patient condition, and proximity to death.

Review Video: Pleural Effusions
Visit mometrix.com/academy and enter code: 145719

Chronic Renal Failure

Chronic renal failure (resulting in end-stage renal disease) occurs when the kidneys are unable to filter and excrete wastes, concentrate urine, and maintain electrolyte balance because of hypoxic conditions, kidney disease, or obstruction in the urinary tract. It results first in azotemia (increase in nitrogenous waste in the blood) and then in uremia (nitrogenous wastes cause toxic symptoms). When >50% of the functional renal capacity is destroyed, the kidneys can no longer carry out necessary functions, and progressive deterioration takes place over months or years. Symptoms are often non-specific in the beginning with loss of appetite and energy.

Symptoms and complications	Treatment
• Weight loss • Headaches, muscle cramping, general malaise • Increased bruising and dry or itching skin • Increased BUN and creatinine • Sodium and fluid retention with edema • Hyperkalemia • Metabolic acidosis • Calcium and phosphorus depletion, resulting in altered bone metabolism, pain, and restricted growth • Anemia with decreased production on RBCs • Increased risk of infection • Uremic syndrome	• Supportive/symptomatic therapy • Dialysis and transplantation • Diet control: Low protein, salt, potassium, and phosphorus • Fluid limitations • Calcium and vitamin supplementation • Phosphate binders

Gastrointestinal Disorders

Cirrhosis and Liver Failure

Cirrhosis is a chronic hepatic disease in which normal liver tissue is replaced by fibrotic tissue that impairs liver function. Decompensated cirrhosis occurs when the liver can no longer adequately synthesize proteins, clotting factors, and other substances so that portal hypertension and liver failure occur.

Signs and symptoms	Treatment
• Hepatomegaly • Chronic elevated temperature • Clubbing of fingers • Purpura resulting from thrombocytopenia, with bruising and epistaxis • Portal obstruction resulting in jaundice and ascites • Bacterial peritonitis with ascites • Esophageal varices • Edema of extremities and presacral area resulting from reduced albumin in the plasma • Vitamin deficiency from interference with formation, use, and storage of vitamins, such as A, C, and K • Anemia from chronic gastritis and reduced intake • Hepatic encephalopathy with alterations in mentation • Hypotension • Atrophy of gonads	• Treatment varies according to the symptoms and is supportive rather than curative as the fibrotic changes in the liver cannot be reversed: • Dietary supplements and vitamins • Diuretics (potassium sparing), such as Aldactone and Dyrenium, to decrease ascites • Colchicine to reduce fibrotic changes • Liver transplant (the definitive treatment) • Paracentesis may be done for palliative relief

Ascites

Ascites involves the accumulation of serous fluid in the abdominal cavity. There are three **types of ascites**:

- **Central ascites** results from compression of the portal venous or lymphatic system from tumor invasion. With this process, there may also be a decrease in plasma oncotic pressure favoring the development of ascites, as a result of reduced dietary protein intake and cancer-induced catabolism.
- **Peripheral ascites** results from deposits of tumor cells on the parietal or visceral peritoneum, functionally interfering with normal lymph and venous drainage. The presence of macrophages also increases capillary permeability and thereby contributes to increasing fluid retention within the peritoneal cavity.
- **Mixed-type ascites** is a combination of both peripheral and central ascites.

Chylous malignant ascites occurs when cancer cells invade the retroperitoneal space causing lymph flow obstruction through the lymph nodes or pancreas. Malignant ascites generally has a poor prognosis. Tumor cells make it difficult to reduce fluid accumulation. Cancers most often associated with ascites include ovarian, endometrial, breast, colon, gastric, and pancreatic cancer. Less common sources include mesothelioma, non-Hodgkin's lymphoma, and prostate cancer.

Bowel Obstruction

Bowel obstruction is a mechanical obstruction of the passage of intestinal contents because of constriction or occlusion of the lumen or lack of muscular contractions (paralytic ileus). In pediatric hematologic/oncologic patients, bowel obstruction is most often associated with non-Hodgkin's lymphomas because tumors may form in the small and/or large intestine (most common), especially Burkitt lymphoma. Bowel obstruction may also occur with hematological malignancies, such as leukemia, and intraabdominal tumors. Symptoms include abdominal pain and distention, vomiting, dehydration, diminished or absent bowel sounds, severe constipation, respiratory distress, shock, and sepsis. Sudden and frequent nausea and vomiting in large volumes, often immediately after intake, usually indicates a bowel obstruction in the small intestines while obstructions of the colon usually result in more delayed vomiting, with fecal emesis. If obstruction is partial or inoperable, dexamethasone may relieve some of the symptoms because it reduces inflammation and swelling and provides relief of nausea. With paralytic ileus, an NG tube may be inserted for decompression. Surgical intervention is used for complete obstruction.

Constipation

Constipation may be caused by primary or metastasized cancers, diabetes, hypothyroidism, hemorrhoids, diverticular disease, neurological diseases, dehydration, changes in toileting, and hypercalcemia. Medications that can cause constipation include opioids, anticholinergics, tricyclic antidepressants, antiparkinsonian drugs, iron, antihypertensives, antihistamines, antacids, and diuretics. Vinca alkaloid chemotherapy also causes constipation by damaging the myenteric plexus of the colon, causing increased contractions without increased movement. Stool laxative/softeners should be taken daily to prevent/treat constipation, especially if associated with opioid use. If patients cannot tolerate oral medications, then methylnaltrexone subcutaneously may relieve constipation. For opioid-induced constipation, reducing the dose of opioid may increase the patient's pain, so treating the adverse effect is more important than removing the cause. Bulking agents should be avoided as they can increase constipation and impaction if the patient is not able to drink adequate fluids, as is common with debilitated patients. While adequate fluid intake is preferred, forcing fluids may increase a patient's discomfort and cause nausea.

DIARRHEA

Diarrhea may be acute or chronic and is often associated with treatment (chemotherapy, radiotherapy) or disease (HIV/AIDS, GVHD). Diarrhea may be osmotic (hyperosmolar preparations/enteric feedings), secretory (chemotherapy and radiotherapy), hypermotile (partial bowel obstruction), or exudative (abdominal radiotherapy). The **National Cancer Institute Scale of Severity of Diarrhea:**

- **Grade 0**: Normal stools
- **Grade 1**: Two to three stools daily but essentially no other symptoms
- **Grade 2**: Four to six stools daily with stools at night and/or moderate abdominal cramping
- **Grade 3**: Seven to nine stools daily with fecal incontinence and/or severe abdominal cramping
- **Grade 4**: >10 stools daily with stools grossly blood and/or fluid depletion results in need for parenteral support

Management may include oral/IV fluids and electrolytes, loperamide 2-4 mg 1-2 times daily, diphenoxylate 1-2 tablets up to 8 times daily, codeine, tincture of opium (decreases peristalsis), octreotide (secretory diarrhea), bismuth salicylate, and clonidine (watery diarrhea associated with bronchogenic cancer). Pectin and methylcellulose may improve stool consistency. Milk products and foods that are high fiber, gas producing, sugary, or spicy should be avoided.

DIABETES

End-stage progression of diabetes may include:

- **Nephropathy and renal failure**: Patients may have recurrent urinary infections, difficulty urinating because of impaired sensation, and progressing to kidney failure and uremia. Some patients may be maintained on hemodialysis or peritoneal dialysis. Others may require catheterization.
- **Retinopathy and vision impairment**: Patients may need orientation to objects about them and vision aids.
- **Peripheral neuropathy**: Lack of sensation increases risks of ulcerations and infections, and some patients may develop severe pain in the feet and legs, requiring pain medications. Patients should be turned frequently with limbs supported and cushioned, and skin assessed.
- **Diabetic ulcers**: Various treatments, including dressings, debridement, and hyperbaric oxygen treatments may be utilized to prevent worsening and promote healing.
- **Gastroparesis**: Patients may have frequent heartburn and feeling of fullness and discomfort. Sitting upright for 1-2 hours after eating and taking metoclopramide may help promote gastric emptying.
- **Hypoglycemia/Hyperglycemia**: Management of glucose levels may become more difficult, especially if the patient is unable to eat adequately, so glucose levels must be monitored frequently, especially to avoid ketoacidosis and hypoglycemia.

Diabetic Neuropathy

Up to 70% of patients with diabetes mellitus develop diabetic neuropathy. **Types of neuropathy** include:

- **Sensory (peripheral)**: Usually bilateral and affecting hands and feet ("stocking-glove neuropathy"). Patients have sensory loss, paresthesias (tingling, itching), and pain (burning, cramping, tearing). Pain usually worsens at night. Foot injuries and ulcerations may occur because of loss of sensation. Some experience hyperesthesia and cannot tolerate any pressure on skin. Patients have increased risk of ulceration and amputation because of loss of protective sensation (LOPS) and peripheral arterial disease (a common finding). Feet should be examined daily, and the patient should not go barefoot. Patients may develop foot deformity (Charcot's foot).
- **Autonomic**: Can affect all body systems, leading to fecal incontinence, diarrhea, hypoglycemic unawareness, neurogenic bladder, gastroparesis, postural hypotension, tachycardia, erectile dysfunction, decreased libido, and vaginitis. Some patients may develop urinary retention and may require intermittent catheterization.

Hematologic Disorders

Neutropenia

Neutropenia refers to an abnormally low blood count of neutrophil granulocytes—the main form of white blood cells and the body's primary defense against infection. It is sometimes also called "leucopenia" in reference to the lack of white blood cells. **Neutropenia** is diagnosed as a polymorphonuclear neutrophil count equal or less than 500/mL. Chronic neutropenia is a sustained condition of minimal neutrophils lasting 3 or more months. Neutropenia may occur from a decreased production of white blood cells following chemotherapy or radiation therapy. It may also occur from a loss of white blood cells due to an autoimmune disease. Neutropenia is silent but dangerous. It leaves essentially no neutrophils to fight any threat of infection. Neutrophils make up as much as 70% of the white blood cells circulating in the blood. Neutropenia can ultimately result in a severe septic situation which can be life threatening. Up to 70% of patients experiencing a fever while in a neutropenic state will die within 48 hours if not treated aggressively.

DIC

The onset of symptoms of **disseminated intravascular coagulation** (DIC) may be very rapid or a slower chronic progression from a disease. Those who develop the chronic manifestation of the disease usually have fewer acute symptoms and may slowly develop ecchymosis or bleeding wounds.

Signs and symptoms	Treatment
• Bleeding from surgical or venous puncture sites • Evidence of GI bleeding with distention, bloody diarrhea • Hypotension and acute symptoms of shock • Petechiae and purpura with extensive bleeding into the tissues • Laboratory abnormalities: • Prolonged prothrombin and partial prothrombin times • Decreased platelet counts and fragmented RBCs • Decreased fibrinogen	• Identifying and treating underlying cause • Replacement blood products, such as platelets and fresh frozen plasma • Anticoagulation therapy (heparin) to increase clotting time • Cryoprecipitate to increase fibrinogen levels • Coagulation inhibitors and coagulation factors

BURN INJURIES

Burn injuries may be chemical, electrical, or thermal and are assessed by the area, percentage of the body burned, and depth:

- **First-degree burns** are superficial and affect the epidermis, causing erythema and pain. Treatment: Soothing lotion, cool compresses, analgesia.
- **Second-degree burns** extend through the dermis (partial thickness), resulting in blistering and sloughing of epidermis with severe pain. Treatment: Silver sulfadiazine, non-adherent dressings, and analgesia.
- **Third-degree burns** affect underlying tissue, including vasculature, muscles, and nerves (full thickness), with no pain because of nerve damage. Treatment: Varies but may include debridement, skin grafts, oxygen, IV fluids/electrolytes, antibiotics, high protein diet, and analgesia.

American Burn Association Criteria	
Minor	<10% body surface area (BSA) 2% BSA with 3rd degree without serious risk to face, hands, feet, or perineum
Moderate	10-20% BSA combined 2nd and 3rd degree burns ≤10% full thickness without serious risk to face, hands, feet, or perineum
Major	20% BSA; ≥10% 3rd degree burns All burns to face, hands, feet, or perineum that will result in functional/cosmetic defect Burns with inhalation or other major trauma

HEAD TRAUMA

CONCUSSIONS AND CONTUSIONS/LACERATIONS

A variety of different injuries can occur as a result of **head trauma**:

- **Concussions** are the most common injury and are usually relatively transient, causing no permanent neurological damage. When the concussion is severe, or multiple concussion occur, however, permanent damage can occur. Concussions may result in confusion, disorientation, and mild amnesia, which last only minutes or hours.
- **Contusions/lacerations** are bruising and tears of cerebral tissue. There may be petechial areas at the impact site (coup) or larger bruising. Contrecoup injuries are less common in children than in adults. Areas most impacted by contusions and lacerations are the occipital, frontal, and temporal lobes. The degree of injury relates to the amount of vascular damage, but initial symptoms are similar to a concussion; however, symptoms persist and may progress, depending upon the degree of injury. Lacerations are often caused by fractures.

Glasgow Coma Scale

The Glasgow coma scale (GCS) measures the depth and duration of coma or impaired level of consciousness and is used for postoperative assessment. The GCS measures three parameters (best eye response, best verbal response, and best motor response) with a total possible score that ranges from 3 to 15. The same scale is used with slight modifications for infants.

Eye opening	4: Spontaneous 3: To verbal stimuli 2: To pain (not of face) 1: No response
Verbal	5: Oriented (Infant: Smiles, exhibits appropriate interactions) 4: Conversation confused, but can answer questions (Infant: crying but consolable) 3: Uses inappropriate words (Infant: Moaning, sometimes inconsolable) 2: Speech incomprehensible (Infant: Inconsolable, agitated) 1: No response
Motor	6: Moves on command (Infant: Moves spontaneously or with purpose) 5: Moves purposefully to respond to pain 4: Withdraws in response to pain 3: Decorticate posturing (flexion) in response to pain 2: Decerebrate posturing (extension) in response to pain 1: No response

Review Video: Glasgow Coma Scale
Visit mometrix.com/academy and enter code: 133399

Classifications of Acute Traumatic Brain Injuries

Traumatic brain injuries may range from mild to severe and may result from impact (falls, motor-vehicle accidents, assaults, or penetration (gunshot and stabbing injuries)). Injuries may be primary with direct assault on the brain or secondary, resulting from hypoxia or hypotension, so initial treatment focuses on maintaining adequate blood pressure and preventing increased intracranial pressure that interferes with oxygenation. TBIs are classified according to symptoms and Glasgow coma score:

- **Mild (GCS 13-15)**: Brief loss of consciousness (LOC), headache, and mild confusion. Recovery is good although some may have persistent symptoms.
- **Moderate (GCS 9-12)**: LOC, confused, focal neurologic defects may be present. Prognosis is usually good, but 12% progress to severe TBI.
- **Severe (GCS ≤8)**: Comatose, severe symptoms, increased intracranial pressure, 20% mortality rate with survivors usually having significant neurological deficits. With severe injuries, patients may require intubation and mechanical ventilation. If injuries are inconsistent with life, patients may become organ donors.

Management of Complications from Acute Traumatic Head Injuries

Head injuries that occur at the time of trauma include fractures, contusions, hematomas, and diffuse cerebral and vascular injury. These injuries may result in hypoxia, increased intracranial pressure, and cerebral edema. Open injuries may result in infection. Patients often suffer initial hypertension, which increases intracranial pressure, decreasing perfusion. Often the primary problem with head trauma is a significant increase in swelling, which also interferes with perfusion, causing hypoxia and hypercapnia, which trigger increased blood flow. This increased volume at a time when injury impairs auto-regulation increases cerebral edema, which, in turn, increases intracranial pressure and results in a further decrease in perfusion with resultant ischemia. If pressure continues to rise, the brain may herniate. Concomitant hypotension may result in hypoventilation, further complicating treatment. Treatments include:

- Monitoring ICP and CCP
- Providing oxygen
- Elevating head of bed and maintaining proper body alignment
- Giving medications: Analgesics, anticonvulsants, and anesthetics
- Providing blood/fluids to stabilize hemodynamics
- Managing airway, providing mechanical ventilation if needed
- Providing osmotic agents, such as mannitol and hypertonic saline solution, to reduce cerebral edema

Spinal Cord Injuries

Spinal cord injuries may result from blunt trauma, falls from a height, various types of sports injuries (especially contact sports, gymnastic, diving), and penetrating trauma. Damage results from mechanical injury and secondary responses resulting from hemorrhage, edema, and ischemia. The type of symptoms relates to the area and degree of injury.

Anterior cord	The posterior column functions remain so there is sensation of touch, vibration, and position remaining below injury but with complete paralysis and loss of sensations of pain and temperature. Injury to the anterior portion of the spinal cord usually results from herniated disks, hyperflexion injuries, or damage to the anterior spinal artery. Prognosis is poor.
Brown-Séquard /Lateral cord	The cord is hemisected resulting in spastic paresis, loss of sense of position and vibration on the injured side and loss of pain and thermal sensation on the other side below level of injury. Prognosis is good. Injury to the right or left half of spinal cord usually occurs from transverse hemisection by knife injury or fracture dislocations.
Cauda equina	Damage is below L-1 with variable loss of motor ability and sensation and bowel and bladder dysfunction. Injury is to peripheral nerves, which can regenerate so prognosis is better than for other lesions of the spinal cord.
Central cord	Results from hyperextension and ischemia or stenosis of cervical spine, causing quadriparesis (more severe in upper extremities) with some loss of sensations of pain and temperature). Prognosis is good, but fine motor skills are often impaired in upper extremities. The trunk area may suffer incomplete loss of sensation and control, and bowel and bladder control may remain intact.
Conus medullaris	Injury to lower spine (lower lumbar and sacral nerves) causes lumbar pain, loss of sensation in medial thighs, numbness and weakness in legs and feet, unstable ambulation, impotence, and lack of bladder control.
Posterior cord	Motor function is preserved but without sensation.
Spinal shock	Injury at T6 or above, results in flaccid paralysis below lesion with loss of sensations and rectal tone, bradycardia, and hypotension.

Signs and Symptoms of Serious Illness

Neurologic Symptoms

End-stage disease progression of neurologic disorders varies, but there are some commonalities:

- **Progressive weakness or disability**: Ambulatory patients may progress to wheelchair bound or bedridden. Patients may be unable to manage personal care or any ADLs, such as eating, toileting, and bathing, without assistance. While range-of-motion and other exercises may help, the changes are usually not reversible, so the caregiver may need assistance to provide care.
- **Speech impairment**: The patient's speech may be difficult to understand or the patient may lose the ability to communicate verbally. Assistive devices such as computerized systems may help, and the patient may be able to communicate through picture or letter boards.
- **Dysphagia**: The patient may choke easily and eventually lose the ability to swallow. Initially, the dysphagia may be controlled through changes in diet (soft or pureed foods) but eventually the patient may need a feeding tube to maintain nutrition and hydration.
- **Respiratory distress**: Positioning and oxygen administration may relieve respiratory distress, but those with severe impairment may require intubation and ventilation.

Myoclonus

Myoclonus is characterized by jerking muscle contractions. Myoclonus is common after opioid administration and mild twitching is usually not of major concern, but moderate or more pronounced myoclonus may progress to seizures. Reducing dosage, utilizing opioid rotation, or changing to an equianalgesic should relieve symptoms in one to two days. In addition to opioids, myoclonus may be associated with AIDS dementia, hypoxic conditions, administration of quinolones, placement of an intrathecal catheter, and neurological impairment following brain surgery. Myoclonus can be very tiring, especially if it occurs nocturnally and interferes with sleep. If myoclonus is very mild, a benzodiazepine (clonazepam, diazepam, midazolam) at bedtime may keep jerking from awakening the patient. Baclofen may also help reduce myoclonus. Protective padding should be placed about the patient (on side rails and assistive devices).

Encephalopathy

Encephalopathy is a degenerative condition of the brain, characterized by alterations in mental status, often with confusion, memory loss, and personality changes. Patients may exhibit physical symptoms as well, such as ataxia, seizures, and tremors. Encephalopathy may be caused by lack of oxygen (anoxic, hypoxic) or disease process, such as infection, liver failure, kidney failure, brain tumors, brain abscess, alcohol withdrawal, vitamin deficiency, (B-1), chemical or alcohol toxicity, increasing intracranial pressure, and hypoglycemia. Management includes identifying and treating the underlying cause as some cases of encephalopathy may reverse with appropriate treatment, which can vary widely. The Glasgow Coma Scale may be utilized to assess level of consciousness. Patients should be protected from injury and oriented frequently. Some patients may benefit from administration of oxygen. Patients should usually be positioned with the head elevated to reduce pressure.

Aphasia

Aphasia is the loss of ability to use or understand written and spoken language because of damage to the speech center of the brain caused by brain tumors, brain injury, or stroke. The speech pathologist should assess the patient and provide guidance in communicating with the patient. There are different types of aphasia:

- **Global**: Difficulty understanding and producing language in speaking, reading, and writing although patients may understand gestures. Use pictures, diagrams, and gestures to convey meaning. Picture charts are useful.
- **Broca's**: Can understand language but has difficulty producing language to varying degrees. Speak slowly and clearly, facing the person, and be patient. Picture charts may be useful to help the patient communicate.
- **Wernicke's**: Difficulty understanding language but can understand gestures and is able to produce language although with some impairment, such as incorrect words or sounds. Patients may be able to write or use letter boards to assist communication.

Dysphagia

Dysphagia may occur in any phase of swallowing:

- **Oral phase**: Difficulty chewing and swallowing, tends to drool liquids and food; food remains in the mouth after the meal.
- **Pharyngeal phase**: Chokes while swallowing and often regurgitates food into the nose during the meal or immediately afterward. Breath sounds and voice may be gurgling after eating because of incomplete swallowing, and patients may feel as though food is caught in the throat.
- **Esophageal phase**: Has reflux and regurgitates food frequently after eating, difficulty swallowing solid foods. Patients rarely cough or choke but may feel as though food is caught in the chest.

If the patient may aspirate, the most appropriate referral is to a speech pathologist. The speech pathologist is able to assess the strength of the mouth, including the lips, the tongue, the palate, and the jaw, and may suggest preventive measures, including positioning, exercises, and diet modifications. In some cases, a feeding tube may be considered or withdrawal of food and fluids in the case of a dying patient.

Comfort Needs of Neurological Patients

Comfort needs of neurological patients include:

- **Physical**: Includes positioning, assisting with mobility, providing assistive devices and training, preventing thirst and hunger, providing adequate nutrition, controlling pain, managing muscle spasms and spasticity or other symptoms, managing bowel and bladder, carrying out skin care, managing adverse effects of drugs, and preventing complications
- **Psychosocial**: Includes helping patient make adjustments to disability, encouraging independence and decision making, addressing depression, reducing uncertainty, providing up-to-date information, encouraging friends and family to participate, helping patient explore sexuality concerns, recognizing stages of grief, being supportive and nonjudgmental, providing patient and family with lists of resources, collaborating with the patient in all aspects of care, and supporting spirituality
- **Environmental**: Includes maintaining comfortable temperature (heat, air-conditioning, blankets, fans), providing adequate light (ambient and artificial), controlling noise, avoiding clutter, maintaining cleanliness, ensuring safety and access (ramps, grab bars, safety rails, shower seats), and ensuring access to transportation

Cardiac Symptoms

End-stage disease progression of cardiac disorders often includes the following:

- **Dyspnea**: Opioids often help to relieve dyspnea. Other interventions include positioning the patient with head of bed elevated, using a fan aimed toward the patient's face, administering oxygen, and avoiding NSAIDS (which may reduce the effects of diuretics and other drugs). If dyspnea is related to pulmonary edema, diuretics and vasodilators may provide relief.
- **Pain**: This may be cardiac or edema-related, affecting the chest or the entire body. Opioids are generally the drugs of choice to relieve pain related to end-stage disease.
- **Fatigue and depression**: Relieving other symptoms and providing both physical and emotional support may help to reduce fatigue and depression.
- **Fluid retention**: Elevating the legs to improve circulation and administration of diuretics and vasodilators (as for dyspnea) may provide some relief.
- **General weakness**: Patients will become bedbound as the condition progresses and unable to attend to ADLs without assistance.

Angina

Impairment of blood flow through the coronary arteries leads to ischemia of the cardiac muscle and **angina pectoris**. Angina pain frequently occurs in males with crushing pain substernally, radiating to the neck and down the left arm or both arms. Females, whose symptoms may appear less acute, may experience nausea, shortness of breath, and fatigue. Stable angina episodes usually last for less than 5 minutes and are exercise-induced episodes caused by atherosclerotic lesions blocking more than 75% of the lumen of the effected coronary artery. They usually resolve by decreasing activity level and administering nitroglycerine. Unstable angina (preinfarction or crescendo angina) is a progression of coronary artery disease and occurs when there is a change in the pattern of stable angina. The pain may increase, may not respond to a single nitroglycerine, and may persist for more than 5 minutes.

- **Nitroglycerine**: Administered sublingually, 0.3-0.6 mg, repeated every 5 minutes up to 3 times. Avoid with myocardial infarction.
    - Adverse effects: May cause headache, flushing, dizziness, orthostatic hypotension, and palpitations.
    - Interactions: Avoid with erectile dysfunction drugs (sildenafil, tadalafil, vardenafil).

Dysrhythmias

Cardiac dysrhythmias include:

- **Bradyarrhythmia** (pulse rates that are abnormally slow because of impaired conduction)
    - Complete atrioventricular block (A-V block) may be congenital or a response to surgical trauma.

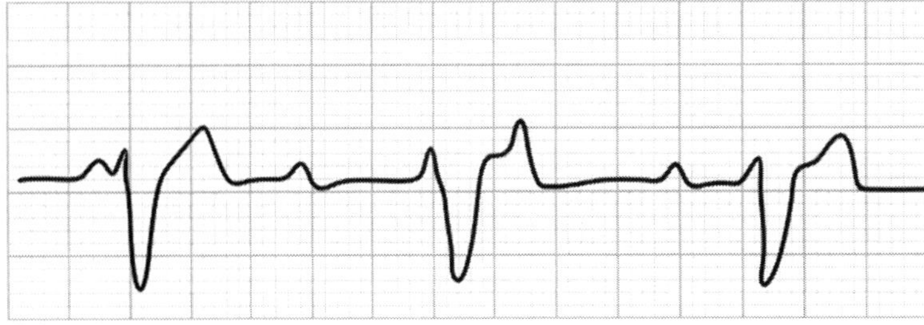

- Sinus bradycardia may be caused by the autonomic nervous system or a response to hypotension and decrease in oxygenation.

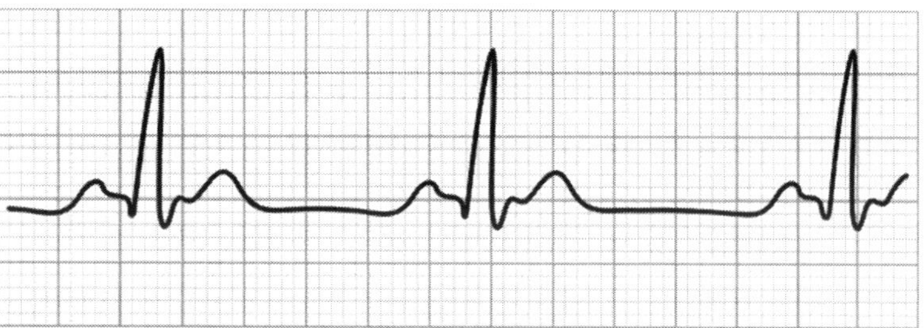

- Junctional or nodal rhythms often occur in post-surgical patients when absence of P wave is noted, but heart rate and output usually remain stable. Unless there is compromise, usually no treatment is necessary.

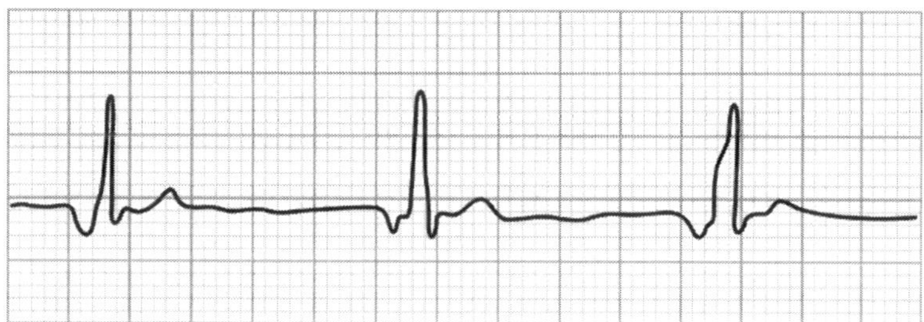

- **Tachydysrhythmia** (pulse rates that are abnormally fast, originating in the atria or ventricles)
  - Sinus tachycardia is often caused by illness, such as fever or infection.

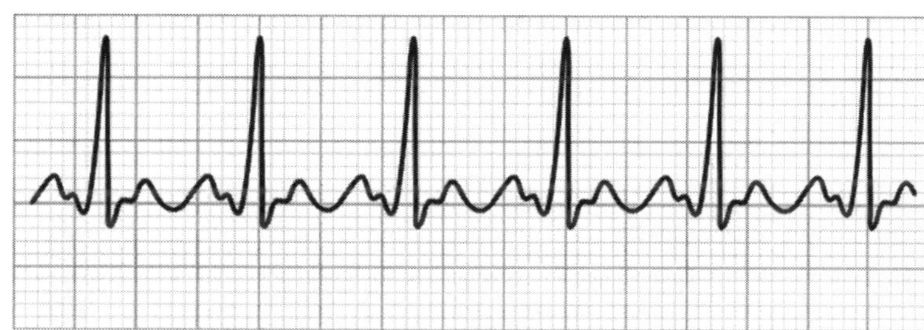

  - Supraventricular tachycardia (200-300 bpm) may have a sudden onset and result in congestive heart failure.

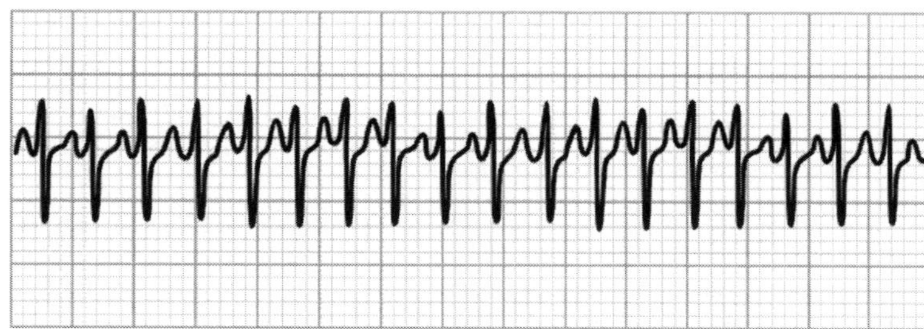

- Atrial fibrillation, atrial flutter, ventricular fibrillation, and PVCs may occur.

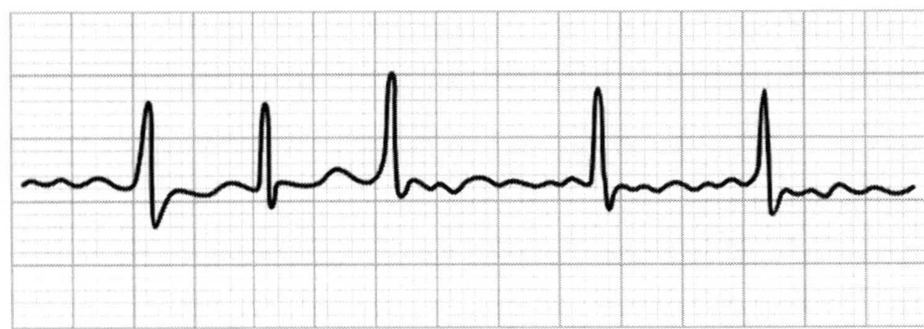

Management of dysrhythmia is usually with medications such as beta-blockers (tachydysrhythmia) or atropine (bradydysrhythmia), cardioversion, insertion of a pacemaker, and cardiac monitoring.

Edema

Edema is a result of excess fluid gathering within the tissues (interstitially). Capillary filtration exceeds lymph drainage, creating a fluid imbalance. The resulting fluid retention causes swelling, decreased skin mobility, tightness, tingling, decreased strength, mobility, and discomfort ranging from aching to severe pain. Skin can change color or even burst from the pressure. Edema is generally assessed according to the pitting scale.

- 1+ edema means the fluid buildup is barely detectable. The depression when pressure is applied is 2 mm and rebounds immediately.
- 2+ edema shows a slight indentation of 4 mm when pressed upon and takes less than 15 seconds to rebound.
- 3+ edema shows a deep indentation of 6 mm when pressed upon that takes 10 to 30 seconds to rebound.
- 4+ edema creates a depression of at least 8 mm when pressed upon and takes more than 20 seconds to rebound.

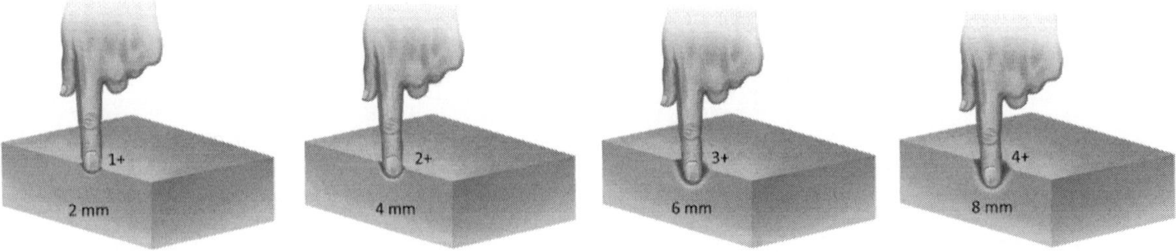

Left untreated, edema can transition to lymphedema. Management usually includes treating underlying condition, diuretics (hydrochlorothiazide, furosemide), elevation of limbs, and good skin care.

PULMONARY SYMPTOMS

End-stage progression of pulmonary disorders often includes:

- **Dyspnea**: Patients with hypoxemia may need supplementary oxygen, and opioids may help to relieve the sensation of breathlessness (air hunger). Patients often breathe more easily with the head of the bed elevated with a fan aimed at the patient's head. Patients may benefit from diuretics (for pulmonary edema) or bronchodilators.
- **Pulmonary cachexia syndrome**: This syndrome comprises anorexia, weight loss, fat and muscle wasting, and weakness. The patient begins to appear emaciated and increasingly frail. Patients may benefit from nutritional supplementation and small, frequent meals. Some medications may improve appetite, such as progestational agents, corticosteroids, cannabinoids, and metoclopramide.
- **Anxiety and depression**: Some patients may benefit from relaxation techniques but others may require medications, such as SSRIs.
- **Cough**: Upright position and cough medicines may help produce some relief.
- **Stress incontinence (associated with cough)**: Patients should limit drinks containing caffeine and may need incontinence products.
- **Chest pain**: Some patients may need opioids to relieve discomfort.

DYSPNEA

Dyspnea is common in hospice and palliative care patients. For patients already receiving morphine, increasing the dose by 2.5 mg may relieve the sensation of breathlessness. Opioid-naïve patients may benefit from 5 mg morphine orally every 4 hours. Providing oxygen (2-4 L) usually only provides some relief if the dyspnea is associated with hypoxia, such as with COPD, although the oxygen may help reduce anxiety. Elevating the head of the bed should be done routinely, but that alone may be ineffective for severe dyspnea. Directing the airflow of an electric fan toward the patient's face may make the patient feel less anxious about the shortness of breath. Cheyne-Stokes respirations are commonly found in dying patients. As the lungs become less effective and more congested, gas exchange is poor, and carbon dioxide levels increase. This increase usually triggers respiration, but as brain function decreases, this function is impaired, so respirations may deepen and then become shallower and irregular with periods of apnea that may last for up to a minute in a repeating cycle.

SLEEP APNEA

Obstructive sleep apnea results from passive collapse of the pharynx during sleep, often associated with narrow or restricted upper airway (micrognathia, obesity, enlarged tonsils). Patients often snore loudly with cycles of breath cessation caused by apneic periods up to 60 seconds, occurring at least 30 times a night despite continued chest wall and abdominal movements, indicating automatic attempt to breathe. ECG changes may indicate bradydysrhythmia during apnea and tachydysrhythmia when breathing resumes. Hypoxemia or hypercarbia may persist during waking hours.

Central sleep apnea involves apneic and hypopneic episodes without obstruction and usually results from cardiac or neurological disorders that cause impairment of ventilation. Snoring is usually mild, and individuals may complain of insomnia because they awaken frequently. Chest wall and abdominal movements do not occur during apneic periods with this breathing-related sleep disorder. Cheyne-Stokes respirations may be present (apnea, 10-60 seconds of hyperventilation, followed by another period of apnea). Treatment for both types includes head elevation and use of CPAP or BiPAP during sleep.

COUGH AND SECRETIONS

Cough is common in patients with advanced heart failure, lung cancer, various other cancers, cystic fibrosis, asthma, COPD, and HIV/AIDS and may be related to infection, inflammation, pulmonary edema, and increased secretions. **Cough** may result from the direct effects of tumors or from treatment, such as radiotherapy. Treatment depends on the underlying cause but may include nonopioid antitussives (dextromethorphan, benzonatate) and inhaled anesthetics (lidocaine, bupivacaine) for non-productive cough. Productive cough is most often treated with chest physiotherapy, oxygen, suctioning, expectorants, and mucolytics. Opioids (such as codeine) may also decrease coughing.

As patients near death, they are unable to cough to clear **secretions** that begin to pool in the oropharynx and bronchi, resulting in rales (death rattles). Because the sound is often distressing to family members, an anticholinergic (glycopyrrolate or atropine) may be given subcutaneously to relieve respiratory distress. A hyoscine hydrobromide transdermal patch is also available, but action is slower, 12 hours compared to 1 minute for injections. Elevating the head of the bed or turning the patient to the side may also relieve rattling.

HEMOPTYSIS

Hemoptysis is the expectoration of blood from the lower respiratory tract. It occurs frequently in patients with advanced cancer due to metastasis or infection. An additional common cause in the United States is bronchitis. The initial assessment needs to distinguish this condition from gastrointestinal and nasopharyngeal bleeding. Patient complaints typically include a persistent blood-producing cough, dyspnea, wheezing, chest pain, fever, night sweats, and weight loss. The severity of hemoptysis is determined by the amount of blood produced within a 24-hour period. Mild hemoptysis is the production of less than 20 mL of blood within that time period. Moderate hemoptysis requires expectoration of 20-200 mL. Massive hemoptysis is 200-600 mL of blood expectorated within a 24-hour period. Massive hemoptysis occurs in fewer than 5% of cases, but it is life threatening and associated with an 85% mortality rate. The primary risk is asphyxiation from blood clots in the airway.

MANAGING RESPIRATORY ISSUES THROUGH THE BREATHES PROGRAM

The **BREATHES program** is used to manage respiratory symptoms in older palliative care patients:

B	**Bronchospasms**	Consider the use of albuterol nebulizers or steroids.
R	**Rales/crackles**	Reduce fluid intake through fluid restriction and discontinuation of IV therapy. Consider using diuretics at a dosage of 20-40 mg/day of furosemide or 100 mg daily of spironolactone.
E	**Effusion**	Determine the presence of a pleural effusion by physical examination and chest x-ray. Treatment options such as thoracentesis or chest tube should be considered.
A	**Airway obstruction**	Assess for aspiration risk and provide preventative measures, such as pureed meals, thickened liquids, and keeping the patient upright during and after meals.
T	**Tachypnea and breathlessness**	Do frequent medication assessments, provide treatments for anxiety as needed. Opioids may reduce the respiratory rate and create feelings of breathlessness and anxiety. Providing cool, moving air may also help reduce feelings of breathlessness
H	**Hemoglobin**	If the hemoglobin is low, consider a blood transfusion.
E	**Education**	Educate and support the patient and family.
S	**Secretions**	If secretions are copious, provide pharmacological treatment.

Gastrointestinal Symptoms

End-stage progression of gastrointestinal disorders may vary according to the type of disorder but may include:

- **Anorexia or difficulty eating**: Patients may benefit from supplementary feedings, small frequent meals, parenteral nutrition, or feeding tubes. Oral foods may require modification, such as in consistency (soft or pureed). Some may tolerate only bland foods.
- **Ascites**: This may result in abdominal pressure and shortness of breath. Patients may need to be positioned with the head elevated. In some cases, paracentesis may relieve symptoms for a short period but fluid tends to recur.
- **Constipation or diarrhea**: Diet modifications (increased fiber and fluids, prune juice) may help alleviate constipation, and antispasmodics or anti-secretory drugs may reduce diarrhea.
- **Bowel obstruction**: Abdomen may become hard and distended. If the patient is not a candidate for surgery, such as colonic stenting, an NG tube may help relieve symptoms temporarily. A venting gastrostomy may be placed to reduce discomfort as well as nausea and vomiting.
- **Pain**: Opioids are often needed to relieve pain, especially associated with bowel obstruction.
- **Nausea and vomiting**: Antiemetics may provide some relief.

Nausea and Vomiting

Nausea and vomiting are common with hospice and palliative care patients occurring in about half of patients with terminal cancer. Asking the patient to do deep breathing and controlled swallowing may help to control the gag/vomit reflex. Other measures include serving cold or room temperature foods rather than hot, restricting intake of fluids during meals, and elevating the head or lying flat (varies with individuals) for at least 2 hours after eating. Patients may benefit from 5 or 6 small meals per day rather than 3 large meals. Fluids should be taken in small amounts (sips) throughout the day rather than in a large volume. Antiemetics are routinely administered to help control nausea and vomiting. Nursing management includes oral hygiene after emesis, control pain, reducing odors, and ensuring clothes are not tight fitting. Other interventions include marijuana, self-hypnosis, relaxation exercises, biofeedback, distraction, desensitization, acupuncture, acupressure, and music therapy.

Bad Taste and Xerostomia

Patients nearing end of life often have a very **bad taste** in their mouths. Strategies to increase patient intake include avoiding highly spiced hot foods and food odors, rinsing the mouth with a salt and soda mixture before eating, using a straw to drink liquids to minimize contact with taste buds, drinking very cold liquids, and eating cold or room-temperature food.

Xerostomia (dry mouth) is a common problem that exacerbates a bad taste and may result from medications, radiotherapy, or disease. Tests to assess xerostomia:

- **Cracker test**: Patient eats a dry cracker. If the patient is unable to chew and swallow the cracker without drinking liquid, the test is positive. Some versions have the patient try to eat 6 crackers in one minute.
- **Tongue blade test**: Tongue blade is placed flat on a patient's tongue. Because xerostomia results in pasty thickened saliva, if the tongue blade sticks to the tongue, the test is positive.
- **Saliva measurement** (stimulated or unstimulated): Mouth is swabbed or patient spits repeatedly into a container for a set duration.

Pilocarpine is a nonselective muscarinic that increases saliva production, but it may result in increased perspiration, nausea, flushing, and cramping. Saliva substitute may provide partial relief.

Intractable Hiccups

Hiccups are involuntary contractions of the diaphragm and chest wall that occur intermittently, usually at a rate of 4-6 per minute. A **hiccup bout** is an episode that lasts up to two days. Intractable hiccups may last indefinitely or recur repeatedly, exhausting the patient and making it difficult to eat, drink, or sleep. Additionally, the jerking motion may exacerbate a patient's pain. Intractable hiccups may be associated with gastric distention (most common), irritation of the phrenic or diaphragmatic nerves, brain tumors, and hyponatremia. Intractable hiccups usually do not respond to the common strategies, which include eating a spoonful of sugar, doing the Valsalva maneuver, and drinking water. Various medications may be used to attempt to control hiccups, depending on the cause: antacids, anticonvulsants, calcium channel blockers, corticosteroids, tricyclic antidepressants, and muscle relaxants. Vagal nerve stimulation through ocular compression, gentle carotid massage, or digital rectal stimulation may be effective in some cases. If the hiccups are associated with diaphragmatic irritation, chlorpromazine 25 mg orally or rectally TID may be effective. In some cases, a cervical phrenic nerve block may provide relief.

Genitourinary Symptoms

Neurogenic Bladder

Neurogenic bladder is bladder dysfunction from lesions of peripheral or central nervous system. Neurogenic bladder may result from stroke, brain tumor, supraspinal lesions, spinal cord lesions, multiple sclerosis, peripheral nerve lesions (diabetes, herpes), Alzheimer's disease, and Parkinson's disease. Nerve damage can cause an underactive bladder that is unable to contract effectively to empty the bladder or an overactive bladder that contracts frequently and ineffectually. **Symptoms** vary:

- **Underactive**: This is characterized by incontinence, dribbling, straining or inability to urinate, and retention. Usually treated with intermittent catheterization. While Foley catheters pose a risk of increased infection, this is not a primary concern in the dying patient, and insertion of the Foley catheter to control incontinence is a comfort measure and may reduce skin irritation.
- **Overactive**: This is characterized by bladder spasms, frequency, urgency, dysuria, urinary tract infection, and fever. Treatment includes antibiotics for infection, absorbent pads, pelvic floor muscle exercises, bladder training, and anticholinergic/antispasmodic drugs (oxybutynin chloride), TCAs, and Beta-3 adrenergic receptors (Mirabegron).

DIAPERS Mnemonic for Causes of Urinary Incontinence

The DIAPERS mnemonic describes the causes of acute urinary incontinence.

D	**Delirium**	Acute delirium and the related confusion may cause urinary incontinence.
I	**Infection**	A urinary tract infection can cause or worsen incontinence.
A	**Atrophic urethritis**	Atrophic urethritis creates irritative voiding symptoms and stress incontinence.
P	**Pharmacy**	Medications such as opioids, sedatives, antidepressants, antipsychotics, and antiparkinsonian drugs can reduce contractility and increase urinary retention, overflow, and stress incontinence.
E	**Excessive urine production**	Chronic disease states such as diabetes mellitus cause polyuria and affect smooth muscle and nerve involvement.
R	**Restricted mobility**	Immobility and restricted accesses to appropriate toileting facilities lead to urinary incontinence.
S	**Stool impaction**	Stool impaction can result in urinary retention, urinary tract infection, and incontinence.

Musculoskeletal Symptoms

Pathological Fractures

Pathological fractures occur as a result of weakening or abnormality of the bone rather than direct trauma. The most common bones affected are the vertebrae, pelvis, proximal humerus, and proximal femur. In the hospice and palliative care patient, pathological fractures most often result from advanced osteoporosis, from bony metastasis (most commonly from the prostate, breast, or lung), and from multiple myeloma or another tumor affecting the bone. Signs and symptoms include acute pain at the fracture site, swelling of soft tissue (sometimes present before the fracture), and muscle spasms. Treatment may require surgical repair (such as femur fractures) or fracture immobilization (cast) to allow healing. Some patients may undergo radiotherapy to reduce cancerous lesions, but radiotherapy may delay bone healing. Patients usually require analgesia and muscle relaxants if they are experiencing muscle spasms. Muscle relaxants include carisoprodol, cyclobenzaprine, or methocarbamol. Patients should have a diet with adequate protein, calcium, phosphorus, and magnesium to promote healing.

Muscle Spasms

Muscle spasms can result in painful cramps, especially in the muscles of the calf. Muscle spasms may result from pathological fractures, dehydration, impaired peripheral circulation, spinal cord injury, neuromuscular disease (multiple sclerosis, amyotrophic lateral sclerosis, Huntington's disease), and electrolyte abnormalities, particularly deficiency of potassium or magnesium. Stroke patients may have muscle spasms on the affected side, with spasticity often occurring within 48 hours, leading to contractures, so range of motion exercises and proper positioning are essential. Numerous medications may also cause muscle spasms, including diuretics (furosemide, hydrochlorothiazide), donepezil, statins, raloxifene, neostigmine, asthma medications (albuterol), and nifedipine. The first step in managing muscle spasms is to identify the cause and determine if that can be modified. Encouraging hydration and stretching the muscles may provide some relief. Some patients may benefit from muscle relaxants and application of heat or cold. Patients with muscle spasms associated with spinal cord injury may have some relief from antispasmodics, such as baclofen, dantrolene, or tizanidine.

Skin and Mucus Membranes

Pruritus and Xerosis

Pruritus (itchy skin) is a common finding in hospice and palliative care patients and may be associated with many different diseases (endocrine, hepatic, neurological, hematological, and oncologic) as well as dehydration, infections, and drugs. **Xerosis** (dry skin) may occur because of aging, chemotherapy, or radiation, and applying a moisturizer may help reduce itching. Most opioids can cause pruritus, but morphine, which causes more histamine release, is more likely to cause Pruritus than other opioids such as fentanyl, codeine, and oxymorphone. If itching is mild, an antihistamine given concurrently may control itching, but in some cases discontinuing the morphine and switching to another drug or rotating between morphine and another drug may be necessary. Application of cold may help relieve itching to a localized area, but heat often increases itching. Topical antipruritics, such as hydrocortisone, may relieve itching but are not practical if itching is generalized. Management depends on the cause and may include propofol, local anesthetics, and androgenic steroids.

Stomas

Stomas may be fecal or urinary and constructed from the small intestine, colon, bladder, or ureters. The stoma should be assessed for color (red if from intestines and pale pink if from ureter or bladder), size, and shape. If the stoma appears blue-tinged, this indicates ischemia. The stoma may protrude at times or retract but should be at or slightly above skin level. Urostomies should have a continuous flow of urine, but colostomies may have intermittent flow, depending on the site of the stoma. The stoma should be carefully wiped clean with water. Superficial bleeding usually stops spontaneously, but severe bleeding may occur with liver disease, anticoagulant therapy, steroid therapy, or a bleeding mesenteric vessel. Other complications may include prolapse, mucocutaneous separation, retraction, stenosis, and direct trauma. The correct size and shape of pouching system is essential to preventing irritation of the skin about the stoma. Peristomal complications can include candidiasis, folliculitis, and contact dermatitis.

Pressure Ulcers

Pressure ulcers result from pressure or pressure with shear and friction over bony prominences. The **National Pressure Injury Advisory Panel (NPIAP) stages** include:

- **Stage I**: Intact skin with non-blanching reddened area
- **Stage II**: Abrasion or blistered area without slough but with partial-thickness skin loss
- **Stage III**: Deep ulcer with exposed subcutaneous tissue. Tunneling or undermining may be evident with or without slough
- **Stage IV**: Deep ulcer, full thickness, with necrosis into muscle, bone, tendons, or joints
- **Suspected deep tissue injury**: Skin discolored, intact, or blood blister
- **Unstageable**: Eschar or slough prevents staging prior to debridement

Patients should be placed on pressure reducing support surfaces and turned at least every two hours, avoiding the area(s) with a pressure ulcer. Wound care depends on the stage of the wound and the amount of drainage, but includes irrigation, debridement when necessary, antibiotics for infection, and appropriate dressing. Patients should be encouraged to have adequate protein and iron in their diets to promote healing and to maintain adequate hydration.

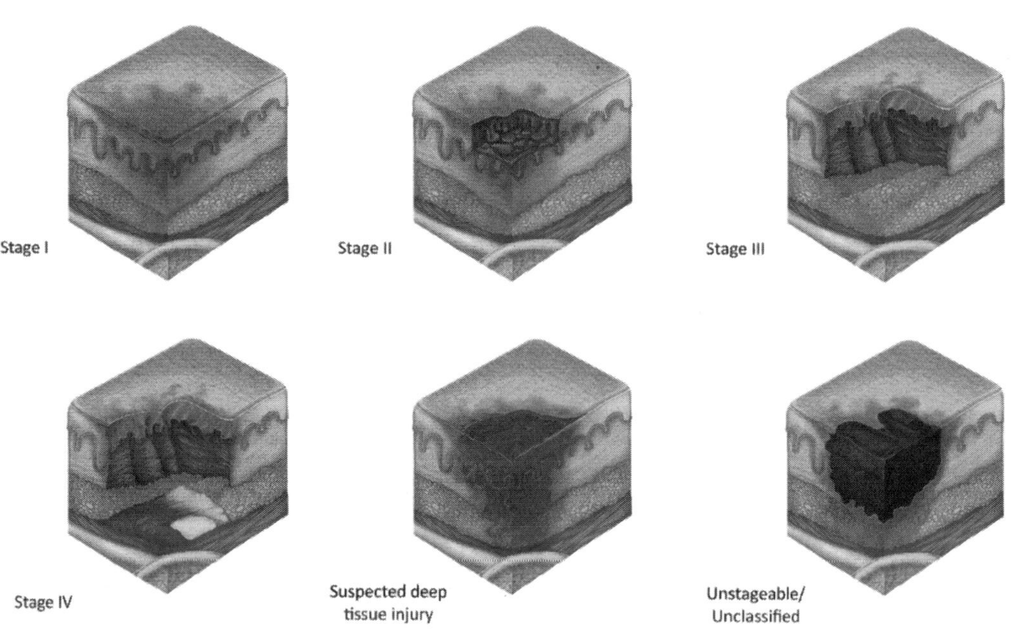

Fungating Tumors

Fungating tumors are those that are rapid growing and erupt in a mass through the skin, often with irregular surface, nodules, and necrotic tissue. These tumors are often very vascular and bleed easily and have copious foul-smelling drainage. They are also often very painful, and the odor is distressing to the patient and family members. Careful irrigation of the wound should be done and dressings applied as necessary. Metronidazole, in gel or solution, has proven to be an effective topical treatment to control infection and odor in fungating and necrotic tumors as it is effective against a wide range of anaerobic bacteria. The solution is used to irrigate the wound, and the gel is applied directly to the tissue. Various treatments (surgery, radiotherapy, chemotherapy) may be tried to reduce the size of the tumor, but healing is unlikely. The patient should receive adequate analgesia to control pain and should receive emotional support.

Mucositis

Mucositis is inflammation of mucous tissue and can occur throughout the gastrointestinal tract as an adverse effect of chemotherapy, other drugs, and radiotherapy. Signs and symptoms usually occur within 10 days of onset of treatment and may persist for 6 weeks or more. The entire mucosa may become inflamed, edematous, infected, and painful:

- Oral inflammation (stomatitis) is common and may result in oral lesions, halitosis, and difficulty eating and drinking because of pain. Good oral care is essential to prevent infection. Special antibiotic or antifungal mouth rinses may be used if infection (such as candidiasis) occurs. Sucking on ice chips or lozenges may relieve discomfort.
- Intestinal inflammation may result in severe diarrhea, treated with antidiarrheal medications, rehydration, and electrolyte replacement.
- Rectal inflammation may result in ulceration, bleeding, and severe pain. Rectal treatment may include steroid suppositories.

Patients who also have neutropenia have increased risk of developing septicemia. Preventive treatment includes benzydamine (for radiotherapy to head and neck) and ranitidine or omeprazole (for chemotherapy). Topical pain relievers, analgesics, and corticosteroids may reduce discomfort.

FISTULAS

A fistula is an abnormal opening or channel connecting two structures. There may be multiple branches from a fistula rather than just one channel. Care strategies include:

- **Skin protection**: Low output fistulas may need only skin barriers and easily changed absorbent dressings. Creases, folds, and depressions may need to be filled with skin barrier paste, wafers, or powder before solid barriers are applied. Solid barriers last as long as they remain intact, liquid skin sealants last up to 24 hours, and skin powders or pastes last up to 24 hours.
- **Drainage control**: If drainage cannot be contained with an absorbent dressing, then ostomy appliances with solid skin barriers and pouches are indicated. The barrier should extend at least 1.5 inches around the perimeter of the fistula. The barrier must adhere to even skin to avoid drainage getting under the barrier, so the opening may need to be enlarged. Pouching systems with barriers that can be cut to fit usually work best. If drainage is extensive, a bedside drainage bag may be used. Very large wounds (more than 4 inches) may require a custom pouching system.

NUTRITION AND METABOLIC CHANGES

NUTRITIONAL ISSUES ASSOCIATED WITH ADVANCED DISEASE

Nutritional issues are a concern with advanced disease. Patients almost always begin to eat and drink less at the end of life, often stopping altogether a few days before death. This is a normal progression, but there is still some debate as to when and if it is appropriate to use tube or parenteral feedings and IV fluids. The decision often rests with the patient or family, but there is little evidence that these interventions improve quality of life or death. Issues commonly associated with nutrition and advanced disease include:

- **Dehydration**: Intake may be hampered by somnolence, nausea, and decreased sensation of thirst.
- **Nausea and vomiting**: Patients may be unable to eat or retain food.
- **Weakness**: The effort to eat and drink may be more than the patient can manage.
- **Bad taste in mouth**: Food may taste metallic or bitter.
- **Xerostomia**: Dry mouth can make it difficult to chew and swallow.

NUTRITION INTERVENTIONS

Generally, the patient receiving hospice or palliative care should be permitted to eat whatever the patient desires rather than focusing solely on nutritional concerns. However, fatigue is a major concern impacting **nutrition**. Education should be provided about the importance of proper nutrition and adequate energy-providing foods when appropriate. It may be helpful to recommend nutritious, high-protein, nutrient-dense foods as snacks and small, frequent meals rather than large meals as well as adequate fluid intake and frequent oral hygiene. Protein supplements may also be suggested. Eggs or protein powder can be added to many foods to increase protein intake. For example, custards can be prepared with double or triple the usual number of eggs without affecting palatability. People with nausea often avoid meat products and those that can cause gas, such as beans. Simply telling patients to eat better is not usually enough to overcome the negative effects of nausea on diet. Chilled dietary supplement drinks, such as Ensure, may be added to the diet if the patient can tolerate them.

Dehydration

Dehydration is common, especially as patients near death. Symptoms are based on the level of dehydration:

- **Mild (5% loss)**: Dizziness, lethargy, reduced skin turgor, dry mucous membranes, and orthostatic hypotension
- **Moderate (10% loss)**: Confusion, resting hypotension, tachycardia, and oliguria or anuria
- **Severe (>15% loss)**: Occurs when total body water decreases but sodium does not; characterized by marked hypotension and anuria as well as symptoms associated with lesser dehydration

Dehydration may result from inadequate fluids, excess water loss, NG suctioning, drugs, diarrhea, vomiting, and fever. Increased fluids may alleviate dehydration in palliative care patients, but patients normally stop taking fluids as they near death, resulting in dehydration and drying of the mucous membranes of the mouth. Frequent mouth care and moistening of the mucous membranes can alleviate mouth discomfort. The mouth may be swabbed with artificial saliva, such as Salivart. As airways dry, secretions lessen, and the ability to cough is reduced. The death rattle also begins to lessen. IV fluids may relieve dehydration but prolong dying.

Anorexia and Cachexia

Almost all patients with terminal cancer or other serious illnesses experience anorexia and cachexia (muscle wasting). In fact, there is little that has been able to reverse anorexia and cachexia when people are in advanced stages of disease, and telling patients they must eat to live only adds to stress. However, some strategies can help to slow the process. Patients often do better when they eat small amounts every hour or two and supplement their diet with nutritional drinks such as Ensure to increase calories and nutrients. The nurse should explore dietary preferences with the patient, trying to find foods that the patient feels like eating, although this can prove challenging and may vary from day to day. Other strategies include lifting dietary restrictions, supplementing food with added protein and calories, avoiding hot food (to reduce odor), accommodating patient preferences for eating schedule and types of foods, allowing alcoholic beverages if the patient desires them, avoiding weighing the patient or stressing weight loss, and never forcing the patient to eat or drink.

ELECTROLYTE IMBALANCES

Sodium 135-145 mEq/L	**Hyponatremia**: <135 mEq/L. Critical value: <120 mEq/L. Causes: Inadequate sodium intake or excess loss, diarrhea, vomiting, NG suctioning, severe burns, fever, SIADH, and ketoacidosis. **Hypernatremia**: >145 mEq/L. Critical value: >160 mEq/L. Causes: Renal disease, diabetes insipidus, and fluid depletion.
Potassium 3.5-5.5 mEq/L	**Hypokalemia**: <3.5 mEq/L. Critical value: <2.5 mEq/L. Causes: Diarrhea, vomiting, gastric suction, and diuresis, alkalosis, starvation, and nephritis. **Hyperkalemia**: >5.5 mEq/L. Critical value: >6.5 mEq/L. Causes: Renal disease, adrenal insufficiency, metabolic acidosis, severe dehydration, burns, hemolysis, and trauma.
Calcium 8.2-10.2 mg/dL	**Hypocalcemia**: <8.2 mg/dL. Critical value: <7 mg/dL. Causes: Hypoparathyroidism and occurs after thyroid and parathyroid surgery, pancreatitis, renal failure, inadequate vitamin D, alkalosis, magnesium deficiency and low serum albumin **Hypercalcemia**: >10.2 mg/dL. Critical value: >12 mg/dL. Causes: acidosis, kidney disease, hyperparathyroidism, prolonged immobilization, and malignancies
Phosphorus 2.4-4.5 mEq/L	**Hypophosphatemia**: <2.4mEq/L. Causes: Severe protein-calorie malnutrition, excess antacids with magnesium, calcium or albumin, hyperventilation, severe burns, and diabetic ketoacidosis. **Hyperphosphatemia**: >4.5 mEq/L. Causes: Renal failure, hypoparathyroidism, excessive intake, and neoplastic disease, diabetic ketoacidosis, muscle necrosis, and chemotherapy
Magnesium 1.6-2.6 mEq/L	**Hypomagnesemia**: <1.6 mEq/L. Critical value: <1.2 mg/dL. Causes: chronic diarrhea, chronic renal disease, chronic pancreatitis, excess diuretic or laxative use, hyperthyroidism, hypoparathyroidism, severe burns, and diaphoresis. **Hypermagnesemia**: >2.6 mEq/L. Critical value: >4.9 mg/dL. Causes: renal failure or inadequate renal function, diabetic ketoacidosis, hypothyroidism, and Addison's disease.

ASTHENIA AND FATIGUE

Asthenia is characterized by loss of strength and weakness, while fatigue is characterized by feeling tired and exhausted after little or no exertion. Asthenia and fatigue are often experienced together in hospice and palliative care patients because of the debilitating effects of advanced disease and chronic pain or as a consequence of treatment, such as chemotherapy and radiation. In some cases, asthenia and fatigue may relate to inability to sleep well at night. The patient should be carefully assessed to determine the cause of fatigue and any aggravating or alleviating factors. Stimulant medications, such as methylphenidate, pemoline, or dextroamphetamine, and methylprednisolone may be helpful for some patients. If fatigue is associated with depression, an antidepressant may relieve symptoms. Treating severe anemia may also relieve fatigue. Fatigue may not be reversible with end-stage disease, but patients should be provided with supportive care and frequent opportunities to rest.

LYMPHEDEMA

Lymphedema is the accumulation of lymph in the soft tissue because of damage to the lymph nodes, such as following radiation or excision. Over time, the tissue becomes distended, hard, painful, and fibrotic. Any limb can be affected, and lymphedema of the arm is common after surgery and treatment for breast cancer. Pressure bandaging and stockings and avoiding dependent positioning can help to reduce swelling and discomfort. With lower extremity lymphedema, there is an increased risk of fungal infection of the toes, so antifungal powder should be applied routinely and the patient should be advised to wear cotton socks and breathable shoes (such as canvas). Signs of fungal infection include redness, itching, and peeling of skin. Antibiotics are given for infections, which are common complications because of stasis and accumulated debris in tissues. Antibiotics may be given prophylactically if patients have repeated infections.

Signs of Imminent Death

Nurse's Role in the Final Hours of Life

The nurse and nursing assistant are important members of the healthcare team throughout the process leading to death, and often develop significant bonds with the patient and family. Many patients and families prefer the presence of a nurse in the final hours of a patient's life, rather than a doctor, because of the close, consistent care-giving relationship. Some patients and families prefer to share those last moments privately. Accept whatever the patient and family choose. The presence of the nurse can be beneficial, as it provides the patient and family with immediate access to a member of the healthcare team who can answer questions regarding the actual process of death. The nurse ensures that everybody has a seat, points out where washroom, telephone, and cafeteria facilities are located, and offers to remain with the patient when family members need a break. If asked to be present, the nurse intervenes only as necessary, out of respect for the family's need for time with their loved one.

The interdisciplinary healthcare team prepares patients and their families for the **imminent death** of the patient. Nevertheless, the actual event is a time of great emotion. *If specific rituals cannot be conducted in a facility because they are against regulations, ensure that the family understands the limitations prior to the death.* Ensure that the patient and family are treated with dignity and respect prior to and after death occurs. Check the patient's vital signs. Record the time vital signs are absent in the patient's chart. If death occurred in a hospice, the nurse pronounces death. If death occurred at home, the CNA or nurse notifies the doctor, who comes to legally pronounce death and complete the death certificate. Do not begin postmortem care until after death is officially pronounced. Offer family caregivers the opportunity to assist in preparing the body if their cultural and religious traditions require participation in postmortem care. The body must be prepared before 2 hours elapse, when decomposition and rigor mortis start.

If it appears death will occur while the nurse is present, alert the family. Assist with contacting family members who are not present, and gathering those that are together. Be cognizant of visitors that are tiring the patient. Close the curtain around the patient for privacy. The patient is the top priority. Encourage family members to enter behind the curtain and speak to the patient singly or in pairs, if this is allowed under the family's customs and they wish to be present. Respect the family's specific religious or cultural observances surrounding the moment of death. If family members choose to remain outside the room, relay information to them as necessary.

Nearing Death Awareness

Nearing death awareness (**NDA**) is a common phenomenon among patients who are dying. When NDA occurs, the patient seems to be aware that death is imminent and may exhibit a sudden change in **mental status**, which may be dismissed as simple confusion. Patients may, for example, begin to talk about going on a journey or taking a trip. Others may say directly that they are going to die, or state a time ("I'm doing to die tomorrow"). Many patients begin to talk about seeing or speaking to someone close to them who has died ("Mother is there waiting for me") or may report seeing angels, Jesus, Buddha, or heaven, depending on their religious beliefs. Some may report a bright light, report a feeling of peace, or report their mind is separate from their body. Others may stare into space and appear to be seeing or listening to something or someone although they can return to awareness if spoken to, so in this sense the experience is different from usual hallucinations. The **Greyson NDE scale** assesses this state with questions in 4 areas: cognitive, affective, paranormal, and transcendental.

ACTIVELY DYING

Active dying, or imminent death, is defined by physical signs and symptoms that indicate likely demise within hours or days. Typically, the patient shows signs of profound weakness, appears gaunt and pale, and the extremities are cool and mottled. He or she lacks interest in food or drink and has difficulty swallowing, which significantly decreases oral intake. Changes in breathing patterns are also common, including shallow respirations with decreased oxygen concentration, dyspnea, Cheyne-Stokes or other irregular patterns, and gurgling or gravelly sounds in the back of the throat from excess secretions. There may be transient improvements in comfort, pain sensation and mental status, but the overall state is one of varying agitation, restlessness, delirium and confusion, increased pain, profound sleepiness, reduced awareness, difficulty concentrating and disorientation to time and place. A semi-comatose or fully comatose state may emerge.

The patient may also experience incontinence of both bowel and bladder. Third-space fluids may gradually be reabsorbed, decreasing the amount of swelling present. The pupils may become fixed and dilated.

FEEDING

A dying patient is not taking in **adequate nutrition**, so his or her metabolism changes and energy declines. When this happens, the patient will have less awake time, which can cause the family concern. Food is often associated with comfort. The family's inability to provide this comfort for their loved one can be a source of distress. The CNA or nurse can assist the family by educating them to the problems a patient may experience by consuming more than desired at this point. The dying patient's altered metabolism means his or her body is unable to handle nutrients in a normal way. Excess food and fluid will cause an increase in respiratory and gastric secretions that can result in dyspnea, abdominal distention, pain, and peripheral edema. All of these conditions put the patient at risk for infection, skin breakdown, and pain.

PROVIDING FLUIDS

Most actively dying patients are **dehydrated** because they are no longer consuming adequate food and fluids, but there is little discomfort associated with this. Dehydration helps reduce nausea, vomiting, and edema for end-stage patients. The most common complaint is dry lips, nasal membranes, and mouth. Oral and nasal drying often results from increased mouth breathing, medication side effects (e.g., antihistamines), and supplementary oxygen delivered by mask or nasal cannula. The family may wish to provide the patient with fluids to drink as a way to relieve suffering and offer comfort. However, the result could be to increase the patient's distress by increasing respiratory and gastrointestinal secretions. Increased secretions lead to dyspnea, abdominal pain and distention, and peripheral edema. A bloated patient is at risk for skin breakdown, infection, and pain. Cleanse the patient's mouth and lips frequently with cool water or protective gel that help them retain moisture, to ease the discomfort without creating more problems.

EDUCATING THE FAMILY

It is often difficult for family members to cope with the physical changes associated with the dying patient. One of the most alarming is significant weight loss and muscle wasting, called **cachexia**. Food is associated with comfort and caring. When asking the family to withhold food, it can leave them feeling frustrated and unable to do anything to help. Reaching this point with the patient may force family members to accept that death is imminent. Educate the family about the physiological changes that take place in the dying patient to help them understand that the withholding of food is actually beneficial. The change in metabolism that results from decreased nutrition causes the body to produce and release endorphins, which are peptide hormones for natural pain control.

Dehydration reduces the production and accumulation of secretions in the respiratory and gastrointestinal tract and reduces edema. It may also decrease pain caused by the pressure tumors exert on surrounding tissues, all of which make the patient more comfortable.

Changes in Bowel Habits

As patients approach death, it is almost universal that their intake of food and fluids decreases. Decreased input means **decreased output of urine and feces**. Monitor the intake and output of patients and be aware of the signs and symptoms of constipation and urinary retention. Constipation, abdominal distention, nausea, and vomiting can indicate bowel obstruction or volvulus (twisted intestine). Urinary retention can indicate kidney failure or a blockage from a stone or tumor. Diarrhea creates significant fluid loss and unbalances electrolytes, which can result in heart attack. Constipated patients are uncomfortable and more difficult to manage. Follow instructions in the care plan for the treatment of constipation.

Congestion

Patients experience **increased respiratory secretions** as they approach death, and are unable to clear them independently. Many experience a drowning sensation. Frequent episodes of coughing leave patients fatigued. Assist the patient with dyspnea to clear the airway by repositioning, and encourage deep breathing and coughing exercises. Use caution, because patients with osteoporosis may fracture ribs if they cough hard. Note the quality of the patient's cough—dry and non-productive, or wet and productive. The RN may suction the airway and ask the doctor to prescribe antihistamines and decongestants. If the patient has a productive cough, the doctor may order the nurse or CNA to assist the patient to collect a sputum sample. The best time of collection is when the patient awakes in the morning, because fluid collects overnight. Wear gloves. Label the jar in ink. Open the sterile jar and ask the patient to expel lung fluid into it, *not saliva*. Cap the jar, place it in a biohazard bag, and refrigerate until pick-up by the lab.

Increased Sleepiness

During the last four weeks of life, end-stage patients experience a marked increase in **sleepiness** due to decreased intake of calories, dehydration, hypoxia, psychological withdrawal, organ failure, and vital exhaustion. As caloric intake decreases, the body conserves energy and shunts blood flow from the periphery to the core to preserve the vital organs (brain, heart, lungs, and kidneys). Rerouting the blood supply triggers the brain to decrease the amount of time a patient is awake. Depending on the underlying disease process, the amount of awake time a patient experiences may be related to a significant decrease in oxygen availability. A low blood oxygen level (hypoxia) will result in sleepiness. For those patients receiving opiates, an increase in sleepiness occurs as a side effect of the medication. Azotemia (also called uremia) causes sleepiness as the kidneys fail. Azotemia causes death 8-12 days after a patient decides to stop dialysis.

Agitation or Restlessness

Patients experience **acute agitation** from urinary retention, constipation, dyspnea, medication side effects, and pain over the course of their diseases. When death is imminent in one or two days, many patients experience another final flare of agitation, which is difficult for families and caregivers to watch. It is the responsibility of the hospice team to monitor the patient for signs of agitation and be prepared with appropriate interventions. The most common cause of agitation in the dying patient is pain. If the patient is nonverbal, rely on physical symptoms to determine when the patient is experiencing pain. Reposition the patient. Monitor for signs that the patient needs pain medication. Divert the patient's attention through music or reading. If the patient approaches death with fear or spiritual unrest, it may express itself as agitation. Ask if he or she wants to speak to a chaplain. Chaplains have contacts among many religions and can arrange visits from the appropriate spiritual leader.

When Death Is Imminent

It is important for the nurse and nursing assistant to understand the cultural and religious beliefs of the patient and his or her family, because these two aspects are highlighted when death is approaching. It is the responsibility of the hospice/palliative care team to support the patient and family and to respect the wishes of the patient. The patient must be monitored for physiological signs that indicate death is imminent, even if the patient does not complain of symptoms. Most patients, within the last four weeks of life, will experience significant fatigue and weakness and require additional assistance. Pain may increase in the dying patient, or the patient's requirement for pain control medication may decrease as the body releases endorphins. Endorphins are polypeptide hormones produced by the pituitary gland and hypothalamus in the brain that act as natural pain suppressants. Most patients experience difficulty breathing (dyspnea) and this is most distressing for families. Careful positioning of the patient and improving air circulation facilitates breathing.

Use of Air Circulation

One of the most common symptoms at the end of life is difficulty breathing (dyspnea). While this can be related to the underlying disease process, most patients near death experience dyspnea as a result of:

- Increased respiratory secretions
- Increased breathing muscle weakness
- Decreased ability to clear respiratory secretions
- Metabolic changes that alter the effectiveness of gas exchange in the lungs

Dyspnea is often the most distressing of symptoms, as the patient fears the sensation of suffocating, and the family is concerned because they are unable to provide relief and comfort to their loved one. The easiest and least invasive way for the nurse and nursing assistant to relieve dyspnea is to use fans to increase the **circulation of air** in the patient's room. Many patients report a decrease in dyspnea when they feel air moving across their faces. If fans are ineffective, inform the respiratory therapist or doctor that supplemental oxygen seems indicated.

Patients' Belief System

Often, patients approaching death feel they have lost control of their lives, which can be as distressing as their physical symptoms. The hospice/palliative care team must understand the cultural, gender, and religious beliefs of patients and their families. **Belief systems** play a vital role in the expectations of the patient and family members. It is also important that nurses and nursing assistants recognize their own personal beliefs surrounding death, and do not impose their own belief systems on the patient and family. Most patients find familiar family and/or religious objects comforting. Treat religious and family artifacts with the utmost respect. Regardless of where the patient is receiving hospice care, he or she deserves to spend time in an environment tailored to his or her preferences. A home-like environment provides comfort and security. Allow the patient to reach the end of life in peace, which will look different for each individual.

The nurse and nursing assistant must accept how the **cultural and religious beliefs** of the patient and family require environmental changes as death nears. They may be required to place particular objects of sentimental value or religious significance around the sick room. The schedule may change to allow for religious rites. They may be asked to assist with ritual washing and dressing.

Some patients prefer quiet and few visitors. If the patient prefers to be surrounded by family and friends, the nurse must rearrange the sick room to ensure the patient's privacy when performing personal care. Support the patient's choice of environment, whether hospice and palliative care is being given in a facility or the patient's home. Develop strategies so that the patient's choices do not interfere with those of other dying patients, such as encouraging the use of headphones. Examine one's own belief systems surrounding death and do not impose personal beliefs or preferences on the patient's environment. Respect the wishes of the patient and attempt to provide the environment the patient desires.

Cultural Influences on Nutrition and Hydration at End of Life

Most cultures attach significant importance to the **role of consuming meals together**. As patients experience the progression of disease and approach death, the goals of nutrition and hydration change. Changing feeding routines often proves distressing for patients and their families. It is the responsibility of the nurse/nursing assistant to understand the changes and help support the patient and their family as the need for food decreases. As death approaches, the goal of eating and drinking is no longer to meet the nutritional needs of the patient. In fact, introducing food and/or fluids as the patient's organs shut down can cause or increase discomfort for the patient. End-stage patients produce increased mucous in the respiratory tract, which leads to dyspnea and the death rattle. If fluids are introduced, the body uses it to increase secretions, which causes increased respiratory difficulty. A more appropriate use of fluid is to moisten the patient's mouth for speaking.

Most cultures attach significant social importance to eating meals together and the hospice/palliative care team must understand the cultural background and the significance of sharing meals in that culture. As a patient approaches death, the goal of eating and drinking becomes social, rather than meeting the diminished nutritional needs of the patient. Anorexia in the patient signals that the dying process has begun. Families often exhibit distress because they perceive that the patient is starving. It is important that the nurse/nursing assistant understands the metabolic changes occurring in the patient's body, and educates and supports the patient and family. Patients who continue to consume food after metabolic changes have started organ shutdown will experience increased edema and discomfort. End-stage patients are unable to process food comfortably, as the intestinal tract slows significantly or stops functioning altogether.

Providing Comfort Measures and Dignity at Time of Death

The nurse should prepare family and friends for the changes they will see as the patient nears death and provide guidance in **comfort measures** for the dying patient:

- Ensuring pain is managed adequately, including medications, such as analgesics and muscle relaxants (if the patient is having muscle spasms), and complementary therapies, such as massage, Reiki, and music therapy
- Providing mouth care with premoistened swabs
- Gently washing and moisturizing the patient's kin with a warm cloth if the patient is cold and cool cloth if feverish
- Talking softly to the patient even if the patient appears to be in a coma and non-responsive
- Accepting and not challenging if the patient appears to be seeing or communicating with deceased loved-ones
- Using FaceTime or Skype to allow family/friends who are not present to participate

After the patient has died, some people will want to spend time sitting with the body and may want to participate in washing and dressing the body, and the nurse should respect their wishes.

Postmortem Care and Services

Postmortem Decomposition

The process of postmortem decomposition begins almost immediately after death. **Livor mortis** occurs as the blood vessels become more permeable and red blood cells begin to break down, resulting in the pooling of blood and staining of tissue that occurs in dependent parts of the body (**lividity**). The skin may appear splotchy within 4-5 hours, but lividity with bluish-purplish-red discoloration is very evident by 5-6 hours. The discoloration remains after compression by about 12 hours and, as red cells break down, a marbling discoloration occurs, and Tardieu spots (tiny dark spots) result from capillary rupture. When lividity occurs, the rest of the body takes on a grey hue. The color of the lividity may vary depending on the cause of death, and the face is often deep reddish-purple in those with cardiac-related death. While liver mortis is occurring, the body also goes through rigor mortis, muscle contracture and stiffening, and algor mortis, cooling of the body to ambient temperature.

Rigor Mortis

Immediately after death, the body tends to be flaccid. However, changes occur within a few hours. **Rigor mortis** is an exaggerated contraction of muscles that occurs 2-6 hours after death when stores of **adenosine phosphate (ATP)**, which is necessary for muscle relaxation, are depleted. Rigor mortis is progressive, beginning with the internal organs and progressing to small muscles in the head and neck (such as the eyelids) and on to larger muscles in the trunk and extremities. Rigor mortis may be more pronounced in those with large muscles while those who are thin and frail may have less rigor mortis. Ambient temperatures may affect the onset and duration of rigor mortis with high temperatures speeding and low temperatures slowing the changes. Chemical activity usually peaks around 12 hours after death and persists for around 18 hours following this peak, but it may persist for another 48 hours or more before the muscles relax.

Algor Mortis

Normal body temperature is about 37 °C, but when body functions cease at death, **algor mortis** (cold death), a gradual decrease in body temperature, begins within approximately one hour, and the body starts to cool by about 1 °C every hour until it reaches **ambient temperature**. The exterior surface temperature cools more rapidly than the internal temperature, and the overall rate of cooling may vary depending on the patient's internal temperature at the time of death, the ambient temperature of the environment, the patient's size (muscle mass, fat), and the presence and thickness of clothing or blankets. High temperatures (internal or external) slow the cooling process. As the body cools, the skin loses elasticity and takes on a waxy appearance. This stage of the process of death ends when the temperature begins to rise again as part of **decomposition**, generally within 24 hours.

Death Vigil

A death vigil entails staying with a dying person and ensuring that the person is never left alone. In some cases, the death vigil may be over within hours, but other patients may die slowly over a number of days, and family members can become exhausted, so they should be encouraged to take turns sitting vigil or to take periodic rest periods. In some cultures, a death vigil means a large number of people are present, but in other cases only one or two close family members. In either case, the nurse and nursing assistant can support this practice by helping to make the room comfortable with adequate seating and encouraging friends/family to maintain a quiet and peaceful environment (low lights, soft music, limited conversation, and distractions). The provider should assist with any cultural traditions that the family desires and ask the family if they want a visit from a spiritual leader/advisor (such as a priest or shaman) and help with arrangements.

Postmortem Care

The body should be prepared in order to provide a clean, peaceful impression for those family members who desire an opportunity to say good-bye before transport to a funeral home. Kindly caring for the body shows respect to the family, the continued value of the deceased, as well as modeling grief-facilitating behaviors for others present. Religious or other rituals the family may find comforting should be encouraged, as should participation in the preparation of the body. Explain the process and what to expect as care is given. Unless otherwise indicated by protocol or the need for autopsy, any tubes, drains, and other medical devices should be removed. Bandages should be applied, as fluids may still be expressed. A waterproof pad or incontinence brief underneath the body is helpful for containing fluids. Packing of the vagina or rectum is unnecessary. Wash the body and comb the hair. Consider dressing the body in something normalizing. It should be noted that the body may "sigh" as it is rolled and the lungs are compressed. If the area is kept cool, the decomposition process will be slowed, allowing the family time to grieve.

Providing Support When Notifying Family and Coworkers at Time-of-Death

The provider should prepare to notify family and coworkers near and at the time of death by asking family members **before death is imminent** who should be notified in the event the patient's condition worsens and how that notification should be carried out (telephone, text) and should post this information prominently in the patient's **chart**. Because of HIPAA regulations regarding privacy and confidentiality, only those coworkers and friends that the patient and/or family have indicated should be notified can be contacted. (Health information remains protected under HIPAA for 50 years after a patient's death). If calling to notify a person of a death, the nurse should prepare the person first: "I'm sorry to say that I have some bad news." Then, the provider should briefly explain that the patient has died, avoiding euphemisms, which may be misunderstood and should answer any questions the person may have. The provider should express sympathy, "I'm so sorry for your loss," but avoid clichés such as, "He is in a better place."

Death Pronouncement

The death pronouncement itself is fairly straightforward, but it can be complicated by the presence of family members or friends, so the provider must remain sensitive to their needs and emotions. Protocols for **death pronouncement** may vary somewhat but generally include:

- Gather information from medical health record and staff members if not present at the time of death
- Identify the patient, verifying patient's ID number
- Description of the body's appearance and location
- Verbal and tactile stimulation utilized and lack of response
- Check of pupillary reflex and finding of fixed and dilated pupils
- Assessment of respiratory status and lack of breathing/lung sounds
- Assessment of cardiac status and lack of pulse noted on palpation and auscultation of apical pulse for at least 60 seconds
- Note and record the official time of death
- Note family and physician notifications
- File report to the CDC for those conditions that require notification if part of responsibility
- Describe notification of appropriate authorities for suspicious death or when regulations require notification of the medical examiner

DOCUMENTATION NEEDED AT THE TIME OF DEATH

Documentation needed at the time of death includes:

- Deceased name, birthdate, address, and unique patient number
- Date and time of documentation
- Reason for attending to the deceased
- List of those present at time of death
- Description of circumstances, including location and complications or disease processes that may have contributed to death
- Outline of death confirmation according to established protocol
- Outcome of assessment and time of death
- Interactions with others present, including staff members and family members
- Specific notifications, such as of spouse, children, or physician
- Description of any special requests or concerns, such as cultural practices
- Discussion regarding organ donation and plans
- Plans for disposition of body (funeral home, autopsy, body/organ donation)
- Notification of medical examiner if required by circumstances/regulations
- Signature, including full name, role, any professional ID number, and contact information

APPROPRIATE CLOSURE ACTIVITIES

When a patient has died, the nurse and nursing assistant should utilize closure activities rather than abruptly ending association with the family, who may have developed a close relationship with the providers involved in their loved one's care. **Closure activities** may include:

- **Make a home visit**: This may be especially comforting to the family of a deceased patient and gives the family members a chance to express their feelings and ask any questions they might have. It also gives the provider an opportunity to help them cope with grief and provide information about resources, such as grief support groups, that may benefit them. The provider should call in advance and schedule the meeting at the family's convenience and should respect their decision if they decline.
- **Telephone**: The provider should call within a few days of death and a week or two later to talk with family members about how they are doing and to see if they have any questions or needs the provider can assist with.
- **Send a card of condolence**: A card and a note about the patient and some specific memory can provide a tangible item of comfort for the family members. A card remembering the patient's birthday and sent at intervals such as 3, 6, 12, and 24 months after death is comforting to family.

INFORMATION AND ASSISTANCE REGARDING FUNERAL PRACTICES/PREPARATION

Some patients or family will have made **advance arrangements** for the care of the body after death (cremation, burial) and a funeral or memorial service, but others may be **unprepared**, so the nurse or nursing assistant should ask the family when death is imminent about whether they have made plans, if the patient has expressed a preference, or if there are any traditional, religious, or cultural practices that they want to carry out and need assistance with before or after the patient's death. The provider should provide lists of local funeral homes and cremation services that are available (with price ranges if available) so that the family can more easily make decisions but should avoid making specific recommendations. If for some reason an autopsy will be scheduled, the family should be advised of when that will take place and how they can claim the body.

Assessments of Specific Populations

Substance Abusers

Assessment of substance abusers (drugs, alcohol) can be met with resistance because of the patient's unwillingness to admit to substance abuse, so the nurse should begin by discussing the importance of the information for diagnosis and treatment. When possible, the nurse should use standardized assessment tools, such as the Addiction Severity Index (ASI), the CAGE tool, and/or the Drinker Inventory of Consequences in order to quantify the presence of abuse. The nurse must remain nonjudgmental and supportive throughout the assessment and should ensure privacy and confidentiality to the fullest extent possible. For example, a patient may not want family members to know about substance abuse. Patients with substance abuse should also be assessed for psychiatric conditions for which they may be self-medicating, homelessness, malnutrition, financial difficulties, and substance-specific illnesses, such as liver disease (alcohol), heart and kidney disease (methamphetamine), lung disease (nicotine), and tachycardia and Parkinson's disease (cocaine). Patients who inject drugs should be assessed for HIV and hepatitis B.

Indications of Substance Abuse

Many people with substance abuse (alcohol or drugs) are reluctant to disclose this information. Common agents include **cannabis** (marijuana), **hallucinogens** (LSD), **stimulants** (cocaine, methamphetamine), **barbiturates** (secobarbital [Seconal], amobarbital [Amytal]), **sedatives** (zolpidem [Ambien], eszopiclone [Lunesta]), **hypnotics/benzodiazepines** (alprazolam [Xanax], diazepam [Valium], lorazepam [Ativan]), and **opiates** (heroin, morphine, fentanyl, oxycodone, hydrocodone). A number of indicators are suggestive of substance abuse:

Physical signs

- Needle tracks on arms or legs
- Burns on fingers or lips
- Pupils abnormally dilated or constricted, eyes watery
- Slurring of speech, slow speech
- Lack of coordination, instability of gait
- Tremors
- Sniffing repeatedly, nasal irritation
- Persistent cough
- Weight loss
- Dysrhythmias (abnormal pulse)
- Pallor, puffiness of face

Other signs

- Odor of alcohol/marijuana on clothing or breath
- Labile emotions, including mood swings, agitation, and anger
- Inappropriate, impulsive, and/or risky behavior.
- Lying
- Missing appointments
- Difficulty concentrating/short term memory loss, disoriented/confused
- Blackouts
- Insomnia or excessive sleeping
- Lack of personal hygiene

CAGE Assessment Tool

The CAGE tool is used as a quick assessment tool to determine if people are drinking excessively or are problem drinkers. Moderate drinking (1 drink a day for older adults), unless contraindicated by health concerns, is usually not harmful, but drinking more than that can lead to serious physical and psychosocial problems. One drink is defined as 12 oz beer, 5 oz wine, or 1.5 oz liquor.

C	Cutting down	Do you think about trying to cut down on drinking?
A	Annoyed at criticism	Are people starting to criticize your drinking?
G	Guilty feeling	Do you feel guilty or try to hide your drinking?
E	Eye opener	Do you increasingly need a drink earlier in the day?

A "Yes" on one question suggests the possibility of a drinking problem while a "yes" on at least two indicates a drinking problem, in which case, the patient should be provided with information about reducing drinking and appropriate referrals made.

Homeless Population

The homeless population has disproportionate rates of mental illness, estimated at 40-45%, many with serious illnesses, such as schizophrenia and bipolar disorder, complicated by substance abuse, so assessment must be multi-faceted, including assessment of substance abuse, nutritional status, functional status, and cognitive status. The need for adequate housing is an ongoing problem with homeless patients. Once released from inpatient care services, the homeless often return directly to the streets or to shelters. They often resist treatment (sometimes not believing themselves to be ill), fail to keep appointments, and lack transportation or money for transportation. They may be victims of violence, have no money for medications, and may not qualify for assistance or may be reluctant to deal with government agencies in order to gain assistance, so referral to social service is often critical.

Cognitively Impaired

Patients with evidence of **cognitive impairment**, often associated with Alzheimer's disease, should have cognition assessed. The Mini-mental state exam (MMSE) or the Mini-cog test is commonly used. Both require the patient to carry out specified tasks:

- MMSE
  - Remembering and later repeating the names of 3 common objects
  - Counting backward from 100 by 7s or spelling "world" backward
  - Naming items as the examiner points to them
  - Providing the location of the examiner's office, including city, state, and street address.
  - Repeating common phrases
  - Copying a picture of interlocking shapes
  - Following simple 3-part instructions, such as picking up a piece of paper, folding it in half, and placing it on the floor
- Mini-cog
  - Remembering and later repeating the names of 3 common objects.
  - Drawing the face of a clock with all 12 numbers and the hands indicating the time specified by the examiner.

Elderly Assessments

Fall Risks

The American Geriatrics Society **Guidelines for the Prevention of Falls in Older Persons**:

- All geriatric patients should be asked if they have had falls in the past year.
- If no falls, no intervention is needed.
- If one fall, the patient should be assessed for gait and balance, including the get-up-and-go test in which the patient stands up from a chair without using arms to assist, walks across the room, and returns. If the patient is steady, no further assessment is needed. If the patient demonstrates unsteadiness, further assessment to determine the cause is necessary.
- If multiple falls, a full assessment should be completed: history, vision, neurological status, muscle strength, joint function, mental status, reflexes, cardiovascular status, including rate and rhythm), postural pulse and blood pressure. Referral to a geriatric specialist may be appropriate.

Risk for Pressure Sores

The Braden scale for predicting **risk of developing pressure sores** scores 6 different areas with 1-4 points. The first 4 areas include sensory perception, moisture, activity, and mobility. The last 2 areas include:

Usual nutrition pattern	Very poor (eats < half of meals; inadequate protein, intake, and hydration) Inadequate (eats about 1/2 of food with 3 protein servings or not enough liquid or tube feeding) Adequate (eats more than half of meals and 4 protein servings) Excellent
Friction and sheer	*(3 parameters only)* Problem moving (skin frequently slides down sheets, needs help to move) Potential problem (moves weakly or needs some assistance, skin slides somewhat during moves) No apparent problem

The scores for all six items are totaled, and a risk is assigned according to the number:

- 23 (best): Prognosis is excellent, very minimal risk.
- ≤16: Breakpoint for risk of pressure ulcer (will vary somewhat for different populations).
- 6 (worst): Prognosis is very poor, strong likelihood of developing pressure ulcers.

Geriatric Depression Scale

The Geriatric Depression Scale is a self-assessment tool to identify older adults with depression. The test can be used for those with normal cognition and those with mild to moderate impairment. The test poses 15 questions to which patients answer "yes" or "no." A score of more than 5 "yes" answers is indicative of depression:

1. Are you basically satisfied with your life?
2. Have you dropped many of your activities and interests?
3. Do you feel your life is empty?
4. Do you often get bored?
5. Are you in good spirits most of the time?
6. Are you afraid that something bad is going to happen to you?
7. Do you feel happy most of the time?
8. Do you often feel helpless?
9. Do you prefer to stay at home rather than going out and doing new things?
10. Do you feel you have more problems with memory than most?
11. Do you think it is wonderful to be alive now?
12. Do you feel pretty worthless the way you are now?
13. Do you feel full of energy?
14. Do you feel that your situation is hopeless?
15. Do you think that most people are better off than you are?

Pharmacological Concerns

There are a number of issues that can affect **gerontological pharmacology** and should be assessed:

- Antidepressants are associated with excess sedation, so typical doses are only 16-33% of a younger adult's dose. SSRIs are safest, but Prozac may cause anorexia, anxiety, and insomnia, so it should be avoided.
- Older antipsychotics, such as haloperidol, have high incidence of side effects. Atypical anti-psychotics appear to be safer with risperidone (<2 mg daily) having the fewest adverse effects. The lowest possible doses should be tried first with careful monitoring of any anti-psychotic.
- Adverse effects of drugs are 2-3 times more common in older adults than younger, often related to polypharmacy.
- Drug and nutrient interactions may impact nutrition by impairing appetite. Interactions may also alter the pharmacokinetics of nutrients or drugs, interfering with absorption, distribution, metabolism, and elimination.

Veterans

Assessment of veterans must include not only the standard assessments appropriate for the patient's age and gender but also assessment of combat-associated injuries and illnesses:

- Shrapnel and/or gunshot injuries: Associated physical limitations, pain
- Amputations: Mobility and prosthesis issues
- PTSD: Extent, frequency of attacks, limiting factors, triggers
- Depression, suicidal ideation
- Substance abuse: Type and extent
- Agent orange-associated illnesses: Multiple types of cancer (including Hodgkin's disease, prostate cancer, lung cancer, and leukemia), Parkinson's disease, diabetes mellitus (type 2), chloracne, and heart disease

Because a large number of veterans are among the homeless population, the veteran's living arrangements should be explored and appropriate referrals made if the patient is in need of housing. Veterans may be unaware of programs offered through the US Department of Veterans Affairs and should be provided information about these programs as appropriate for the patient's needs.

Financial Assistance

Financial Issues

Even with insurance and Medicare, patients may incur huge medical costs for medications alone, and if they need nursing care at home or in a facility, the costs can range from $6,000 to over $12,000 monthly, quickly depleting savings. Medicare strictly limits hospital and extended care stay as well as home health care. When a patient is no longer improving, such as with terminal illness or Alzheimer's disease, their care is not paid for until they are eligible for hospice care, and that has limitations too. Long-term care is not provided by Medicare or most insurance policies unless the insurance is especially intended for that purpose, and these policies are costly. This leaves patients and families with financial burdens that they sometimes cannot pay.

Financial Assistance Organizations

Numerous local, state, and national **organizations** are available to provide hospice and palliative care patients with financial assistance. Organizations include:

- **Patient Advocate Foundation**: Provides assistance for co-pays and transportation expenses for cancer patients and has aid programs specifically for those with metastatic breast cancer and multiple myeloma.
- **Partnership for Prescription Assistance**: Provides information about free or low-cost prescription drugs.
- **PAN Foundation**: Offers financial assistance to pay medical costs through 60 disease-specific programs.
- **Healthwell Foundation**: Provides financial assistance through the Emergency Cancer Relief Fund.
- **CancerCare**: Has a financial assistance program that assists with costs of transportation, home care, child care, and co-payments. Breast cancer patients can receive financial assistance for medications, lymphedema supplies, and durable medical supplies.
- **The Samfund**: Provides twice yearly grants to assist young (21-39) cancer patients with living expenses, tuition, education, medical bills, and various other health-related expenses.

Providing Cost-Effective Quality Care

It's important for the nurse to consider not only the cost-benefit (savings) of interventions but also the cost-effectiveness. A **cost-benefit analysis** uses average cost of problem (such as infection) and the cost of intervention to demonstrate savings. A cost-effective analysis, on the other hand, measures the effectiveness of an intervention rather than directly measuring the monetary savings. Each year, about 2 million nosocomial infections result in 90,000 deaths and an estimated $6.7 billion in additional health costs. From that perspective, decreasing infections should reduce costs, but there are human savings in suffering as well, and it can be difficult to place a dollar value on that. If each infection adds about 12 days to hospitalization, then a reduction in infection by 5 would be calculated as $5 \times 12 = 60$ fewer patient infection days and increased health and wellbeing.

Community Resources Helpful for Hospice or Palliative Care Patient

Community resources that may be helpful for the hospice or palliative care patient include:

- **Home health agencies**: These can provide homebound patients with medical treatment, monitoring, and personal care (bathing) and referral to other needed services, such as a social worker.
- **Volunteer agencies**: These vary but may include faith-based or other volunteers who will visit, assist with shopping and/or cooking, transport patients, sit with patients, or carry out other non-skilled activities to support the patient and family.
- **Medical supply companies**: Patients may need a wide variety of assistive devices, including small items such as grab/reach tools, tub rails, and grab bars, and larger devices, such as wheelchairs, walkers, lifts, and hospital beds.
- **Educational resources**: These may include libraries (medical and general), podcasts, videos, national organizations (such as the Alzheimer's Association), and internet sources.
- **Support groups**: Local hospitals, senior centers, and organizations often provide a variety of support groups for both patients and family/caregivers, such as support groups for those with cancer.
- **Meal programs**: Home meal delivery may be necessary.

Community/Internet Resources Available to Support Patients and Families

Community/internet resources available to support patients and their families include:

- **Association of Cancer Online Resources (ACOR)**: Provides information and internet support groups for patients and families as well as information about diseases and treatment.
- **American Cancer Society**: Provides support groups and assistance with non-medical expenses, such as durable medical equipment, transportation costs, and hair replacement wigs. The "Look Good, Feel Better" program provides assistance with techniques to minimize physical changes caused by treatment.
- **Group Loop**: Provides an online support group for teens living with cancer including discussion boards, personal blogs, and video journals.
- **National Children's Cancer Society (NCCS)**: Provides financial assistance for non-medical expenses.
- **Ronald McDonald House**: Provides living accommodations for families, care mobiles, and family rooms (in hospitals).
- **Sibshops**: Provides workshops for siblings.
- **Songs of Love Foundation**: Provides free personalized songs for children and teens with severe illness.
- **Starlight Foundation**: Provides personalized entertainment experiences for children with life-threatening illness.
- **13Thirty Cancer Connect**: Provides online support for teens and young adults
- **CancerCare**: Provides limited financial assistance (transportation costs, co-payments), information about managing costs, and links to various resources.

Identifying Past and Present Goals and Expectations

When collaborating with the patient and family, the nurse should begin by educating the patient and family about patient rights and asking what **goals and expectations** they have. In order to develop the plan of care, the nurse must know what the patient and family desire, keeping in mind that goals may change. For example, if a patient's goal is to remain mentally alert until death, this may affect the plan for managing pain. If a desired outcome is that the patient die in the home, then the plan of care must include the resources needed to facilitate this. The nurse should ask that the patient and caregiver or other family members list the goals and outcomes that are most important to them and then should compare and discuss the items as they may not always be in agreement. Some negotiation and discussion may be required. While a patient may want to remain at home, for example, the caregiver may prefer that the patient be hospitalized.

Health Beliefs and Traditions Regarding Death

Individual beliefs and traditions regarding death vary widely, and these can affect how the patient and family deal with the end of life. The nurse should discuss these issues with the patient and/or family in order to ensure their needs are met. Those with strong spiritual beliefs may want spiritual advisors (priests, shamans, ministers, monks) present to provide support or perform rituals. People who have no belief in an afterlife may face death with resolution or may be frightened at the thought of the total end of their existence. Those who believe in reincarnation may find comfort in the thought of their rebirth but may also fear karma for the mistakes they made in this life. Some may feel that they will be in a loving place after death while others fear they will suffer torment for their sins. The nurse should remain supportive and allow patients and families to express their feelings, fears, and concerns.

Intervention and Management

Diagnostic Tests and Procedures

Colorectal Screening

Recommendations for **colorectal screening** are based on age and risk:

- Age 50 with average risk (patient is asymptomatic without risk factors).
- Age 40 with increased risk (patient has a family history of colorectal cancer in first or second-degree relatives, family history of genetic syndrome (FAP, HNLPCC), adenomatous polyps in first-degree relatives before age 6, history of polyps or colorectal cancer, or history of inflammatory bowel disease).
- Screening should continue through age 75, after which the benefit of this intervention decreases.

Fecal occult blood	Yearly: checks for blood in stool.
Flexible sigmoidoscopy	Every 5 years: Scope to check for polyps or signs of cancer in rectum and lower third of colon (often done with fecal occult blood test).
Colonoscopy	Every 10 years or as follow-up for abnormalities in other screening: Longer flexible scope, usually with anesthesia, to check rectum and entire colon. It allows for removal of polyps and small cancerous lesions. It also allows for biopsies and provides surveillance of inflammatory bowel disease.
CT (Virtual) colonoscopy	Every 5 years: CT scan (with contrast unless contraindicated) to visualize intestinal abnormalities.

Osteoporosis Screening

The United States Preventive Task Force recommends all people, especially women ≥65 years, be screened for **osteoporosis** and those with increased risk factors from age 60. Risk factors include:

F	**Fractures**	Family history of osteoporotic fractures. Personal history of vertebral or hip fractures.
R	**Race**	Asians and Caucasians have the highest risk.
A	**Age and gender**	Women over age 65 have the highest risk.
C	**Chronic disease/medications**	Diabetes, Addison's disease, Cushing's disease, inflammatory bowel disease, eating disorders, hyperparathyroidism. Medications, such as corticosteroids, excess thyroid medication, and chemotherapy drugs may increase risk.
T	**Thin bones, low weight**	Weight <134 pounds.
U	**Underactivity**	Inadequate exercise.
R	**Reduced estrogen**	Post-menopausal.
E	**Excessive alcohol intake and smoking**	Alcohol disrupts calcium balance and impairs vitamin D metabolism. Smoking has an anti-estrogen effect.
D	**Diet**	Inadequate calcium and vitamin D.

Screening is per a bone density test, usually a DEXA scan. Results are expressed as a T-score. A -2.0 score is the beginning point for osteoporosis: 0–10 = normal, -1.0 = 10% below normal, -2.0 = 20% below normal.

Lung Cancer Screening

Routine screening for **lung cancer** in the absence of symptoms is not recommended because chest x-rays and sputum cytology have not proven effective at early diagnosis. Repeated exposure to radiation increases risk of cancer although screening may be done if secondary lung cancer is a risk:

Risk factors	Signs and symptoms
Any history of smoking (cigarettes, marijuana, crack cocaine)	Hemoptysis
Exposure to second-hand smoke	Dyspnea
Exposure to environmental toxins (asbestos, radon, chemicals)	Persistent cough
Family history of lung or GU cancer	Recurrent bronchitis/pneumonia
Previous cancer	Clubbing

If symptoms occur, screening tests may include spirometry, chest x-ray, and spiral CT scan (which is most effective at identifying small lesions). CT scan cannot differentiate cancer from other lesions, such as scar tissue or infection, so when small lesions are evident, a course of antibiotics may be given to determine if the lesions resolve. Repeat CT may be done to determine if the lesion is growing (an indication of cancer). Screening recommendations have not yet been established although clinical trials are in progress to determine the efficacy of different protocols.

Breast Cancer Screening

The US Preventative Services Task Force recommends monthly breast self-exams for all women and screening mammograms every 1-2 years for all women ages ≥50. Women who are at increased risk for breast cancer may be advised to have mammograms prior to age 40, but breast tissue is denser and mammograms are less accurate. Risk factors include:

- Previous breast cancer
- Family history of breast cancer
- Genetic alterations (BRCA1, BRCA2)
- Early onset of periods (<12) or late menopause (>55)
- Long-term hormonal replacement therapy (HRT) of >5 years
- History of obesity, alcoholism, low activity
- Post-radiation therapy
- History of taking diethylstilbestrol (DES)
- Highly dense breasts

Both false positives and false negatives can occur. Any positive result should be verified by diagnostic mammogram, ultrasound, biopsy, MRI, or PET.

Prostate Cancer Screening

While screening for **prostate cancer** is generally recommended for men annually after age 50, there is not yet a specific screening recommendation or a consensus of medical opinion about screening due to the risks involved with the prostate specific antigen (PSA) test in particular. The current consensus is that the conversation regarding prostate cancer screening should begin with men at age 50. Physicians should provide the appropriate information in order for the patient to make an informed decision on whether to get screened. Men who have a close family member with prostate cancer (father, brother) or who are African American are at increased risk and may be advised to have screening earlier. The two tests that are routinely done are the digital rectal exam (DRE) to palpate the size of the prostate and to note any abnormalities. The other test is PSA test.

The PSA level tends to increase with age and prostate problems, but many other factors can cause the PSA level to increase. PSA <4 is usually considered within normal range. Risks involved with the PSA test include false positives (leading to overdiagnosis, psychological stress, and additional invasive procedures) and physical complications. Additionally, prostate cancers tend to grow slowly and may have little impact on a man's life while surgery can lead to impotence and/or incontinence. If screening indicates the possibility of cancer, further tests, such as a transrectal ultrasound and biopsy may be done.

Laboratory Tests to Evaluate Red Blood Cells

Laboratory tests to evaluate **red blood cells** include:

Total RBCs	Females >18 years: 4.0–5.0 million per mm^3 Males >18 years: 4.5–5.5 million per mm^3
Hemoglobin	Red blood cells (RBCs or erythrocytes) are biconcave disks that contain hemoglobin (95% of mass), which carries oxygen throughout the body. The heme portion of the cell contains iron, which binds to the oxygen. RBCs live about 120 days after which they are destroyed and their hemoglobin is recycled or excreted. Females >18 years: 12.0–16.0 g/dL Males >18 years: 14.0–17.46 g/dL
Hematocrit	Indicates the proportion of RBCs in a liter of blood (usually about 3 times the hemoglobin number). Normal values: Females >18 years: 36–48% Males >18 years: 45–52%
Mean corpuscular volume (MCV)	MCV values indicate the size of RBCs and can differentiate types of anemia. For adults, <80 is microcytic and >100 is macrocytic. Normal values: Females >18 years: 76–96 μm^3 Males > 18 years: 84–96 μm^3
Reticulocyte count	Measures marrow production and should rise with anemia. Normal values: 0.5–1.5% of total RBCs

WBC Count and Differential

White blood cell (leukocyte) count is used as an indicator of bacterial and viral infection. WBC count is reported as the total number of all white blood cells.

- Normal WBC count for adults: 4,800–10,000
- Acute infection: 10,000+, 30,000 indicates a severe infection
- Viral infection: 4,000 and below

The **differential** provides the percentage of each different type of leukocyte. An increase in the white blood cell count is usually related to an increase in one type and often an increase in immature neutrophils, known as bands. This is commonly referred to as a "shift to the left," an indication of an infectious process.

Cells	Normal value	Changes
Immature neutrophils (bands)	1–3%	Increase with infection
Segmented neutrophils (segs)	50–62%	Increase with acute, localized, or systemic bacterial infections
Eosinophils	0–3%	Decrease with stress and acute infection
Basophils	0–1%	Decrease during acute stage of infection
Lymphocytes	25–40%	Increase in some viral and bacterial infections
Monocytes	3–7%	Increase during recovery stage of acute infection

GLUCOSE AND HEMOGLOBIN A1C LABORATORY TESTS

Glucose is manufactured by the liver from ingested carbohydrates and is stored as glycogen for use by the cells. If intake is inadequate, glucose can be produced from muscle and fat tissue, leading to increased wasting. High levels of glucose are indicative of diabetes mellitus (the inability of the pancreas to secrete ample insulin to deliver glucose to the cells. Diabetes mellitus predisposes people to skin injuries, sloe healing, and infection. Fasting blood glucose levels are used to diagnose and monitor diabetes, but many factors (stress, diet, disease) may impact glucose levels:

- Normal values: 70–99 mg/dL
- Impaired: 100–125 mg/dL
- Diabetes: ≥126 mg/dL

The **hemoglobin A1c** (HbA1c) test provides the average glucose concentration in the blood. Red blood cells survive about 120 days and are exposed to plasma glucose. These glucose molecules combine with hemoglobin A to form glycated hemoglobin. The percentage of glucose found in the hemoglobin represents average glucose levels over a 3-month period, a more reliable indicator of blood glucose levels than the fasting blood glucose.

- Normal value: <6% (6 = 135 blood glucose)
- Elevation: >7% (7 = 170 blood glucose)

COAGULATION PROFILE

The coagulation profile measures clotting mechanisms, identifies clotting disorders, screens preoperative patients, and diagnoses excessive bruising and bleeding. Values vary depending on lab:

Prothrombin time (PT)	10–14 seconds	Increases with anticoagulation therapy, vitamin K deficiency, decreased prothrombin, DIC, liver disease, and malignant neoplasm. Some drugs may shorten PT.
Partial thromboplastin time (PTT)	30–45 seconds	Increases with hemophilia A and B, von Willebrand disease, vitamin deficiency, lupus, DIC, and liver disease.
Activated partial thromboplastin time (aPTT)	21–35 seconds	Similar to PTT, but decreases in extensive cancer, early DIC, and after acute hemorrhage. Used to monitor heparin dosage.
Thrombin clotting time (TCT) or Thrombin time (TT)	7–12 seconds (<21)	Used most often to determine the dosage of heparin. Prolonged with multiple myeloma, abnormal fibrinogen, uremia, and liver disease.
Bleeding time	2–9.5 minutes	(Using the IVY method on the forearm) Increases with DIC, leukemia, renal failure, aplastic anemia, von Willebrand disease, some drugs, and alcohol.
Platelet count	150,000–400,000	Increased bleeding <50,000 and increased clotting >750,000.

Review Video: The Coagulation Profile
Visit mometrix.com/academy and enter code: 423595

ENDOCRINE HORMONE FUNCTION STUDIES

Endocrine hormone function studies include:

Pituitary gland	Serum levels of pituitary hormones and hormones of target organs, dependent on stimulation by pituitary hormones, are measured to determine abnormalities.
Thyroid gland	**Thyroid stimulating hormone (TSH)** (0.4–6.15 mIU/L). Increase in TSH indicates hypothyroidism and decrease indicates hyperthyroidism **Free thyroxine (FT_4)** (0.9–1.7 ng/dL). FT_4 is used to confirm TSH abnormalities. **Serum T_3** (75–195 ng/dL) and **T_4** (4.5–11.5 μg/dL). These usually increase together, but increases in T_3 more accurately diagnoses hyperthyroidism. **T_3 resin uptake** (25-35%). Increases with hyperthyroidism and decreases with hypothyroidism.
Parathyroid gland	**Parathormone level** (20-70 mEq/L) and **serum calcium** levels (1.15-1.34 mg/dL). Both increase with hyperparathyroidism. Calcium level decreases with hypoparathyroidism and phosphate levels (2.4-4.1 mEq/L to 6 mEq/L) increase.
Adrenal gland	**Catecholamine (urine and serum) levels**: Epinephrine (100 pg/mL) and norepinephrine (<100-550 pg/mL) elevate with pheochromocytoma. Electrolyte and glucose levels. ACTH and serum cortisol levels and ACTH stimulation test to evaluate for Addison's. Dexamethasone suppression test for Cushing's disease.

LIVER FUNCTION STUDIES

Liver function studies include:

Bilirubin	Determines the ability of the liver to conjugate and excrete bilirubin: **Direct** 0.0–0.3 mg/dL, **Total** 0.0–0.9 mg/dL, and **Urine** 0
Total protein	Determines if the liver is producing protein in normal amounts: 7.0–7.5 g/dL **Albumin**: 4.0–5.5 g/dL **Globulin**: 1.7–3.3 g/dL Serum protein electrophoresis is done to determine the ratio of proteins. **Albumin/globulin (A/G) ratio**: 1.5:1 to 2.5:1 (Albumin should be greater than globulin.)
Prothrombin time (PT)	100% or clot detection in 10 to 14 seconds. PT increased with liver disease. **International normalized ratio (INR)** (PT result/normal average): <2 for those not receiving anticoagulation and 2.0 to 3.0 those receiving anticoagulation. Critical value: >3 in patients receiving anticoagulation therapy.
Alkaline phosphatase	17–142 in adults. (Normal values vary with method.) Indicates biliary tract obstruction if no bone disease.
AST (SGOT)	10–40 units. (Increases in liver cell damage.)
ALT (SGPT)	5–35 units. (Increases in liver cell damage.)
GGT, GGTP	5–55 µ/L in females, 5-85 µ/L in males. (Increases with alcohol abuse.)
LDH	100–200 units. (Increases with alcohol abuse.)
Serum ammonia	150–250 mg/dL (Increases in liver failure.)
Total Cholesterol	Normal: <200. Increases with bile duct obstruction and decreases with parenchymal disease.

RENAL FUNCTION STUDIES

Renal function studies include:

Specific gravity	1.015–1.025. Determines a kidney's ability to concentrate urinary solutes.
Osmolality (urine)	350–900mOsm/kg/24 hours. Shows early defects if the kidney's ability to concentrate urine is impaired.
Osmolality (serum)	275–295 mOsm/kg.
Uric acid	Males 4.4–7.6, Females 2.3–6.6. Levels increase with renal failure.
Creatinine clearance (24-hour)	Males 85–125 mL/min/1.73 m^2, Females 75–115 mL/min/1.73 m^2. Evaluates the amount of blood cleared of creatinine in 1 minute. Approximates the glomerular filtration rate.
Serum creatinine	0.6–1.2mg/dL. Increases with impaired renal function, urinary tract obstruction, and nephritis. Level should remain stable with normal functioning.
Urine creatinine	Males 14–26 mg/kg/24 hr, Females 11–20 mg/kg/24 hr.
Blood urea nitrogen (BUN)	7–8 mg/dL (8–20 mg/dL >age 60). Increase indicates impaired renal function, as urea is the end product of protein metabolism.
BUN/creatinine ratio	10:1. Increases with hypovolemia. With intrinsic kidney disease, the ratio is normal, but the BUN and creatinine are increased.

URINALYSIS

Urinalysis evaluates:

Color	Pale yellow/amber and darkens when urine is concentrated or other substances (such as blood or bile) are present.
Appearance	Should be clear but may be slightly cloudy.
Odor	Should be slight. Bacteria may give urine a foul smell, depending upon the organism.
Specific gravity	1.015–1.025. May increase if protein levels increase or if there is fever, vomiting, or dehydration.
pH	Usually in the 4.5–8 range with an average of 5–6.
Sediment	Red cell casts from acute infections, broad casts from kidney disorders, and white cell casts from pyelonephritis. Leukocytes >10/mL are present with urinary tract infections.
Glucose, ketones, protein, blood, bilirubin, and nitrate	Should all be negative. Urine glucose may increase with infection (with normal blood glucose). Frank blood may be caused by some parasites and diseases but also by drugs, smoking, excessive exercise, and menstrual fluids. Increased red blood cells may result from lower urinary tract infections.
Urobilinogen	0.1–1.0 units.

DETERMINING PROGNOSIS

Prognosis is based on a review of many different factors:

- **Evidence**: This includes laboratory results, pathology reports, and other measures that provide information about diagnosis and the stage/grade or seriousness of the disease.
- **Surgical procedure/observation**: This includes the type of procedure and the extent to which the problem is resolved, such as complete or partial removal of a tumor, or open-and-close.
- **Age of patient**: Younger patients generally have a stronger immune system and heal more easily than older adults.
- **General health**: Those with generally good health may have more physical reserves than those already in a weakened condition because of disease.
- **Resilience**: Some patients have a better coping ability and tend to recover more quickly for illness.
- **Support system**: A strong support system is important for follow-up and adherence to treatment protocols.
- **Survival statistics**: These include average life expectancies for different diseases, such as breast cancer, based on numerous studies.

OUTCOMES EVALUATION

Outcomes evaluation is an important component of evidence-based practice, which involves both internal and external research, and is important when modifying the plan of care. All treatments are subjected to review to determine if they produce positive outcomes, and policies and protocols for outcomes evaluation should be in place. **Outcomes evaluation** includes the following:

- Monitoring over the course of treatment involves careful observation and record keeping that notes progress, with supporting laboratory and radiographic evidence as indicated by condition and treatment.

- Evaluating results includes reviewing records as well as current research to determine if outcomes are within acceptable parameters.
- Sustaining involves continuing treatment, but continuing to monitor and evaluate.
- Improving means to continue the treatment but with additions or modifications in order to improve outcomes.
- Replacing the treatment with a different treatment must be done if outcomes evaluation indicates that current treatment is ineffective.

Change in Level of Care

Advocating for the hospice and palliative care patient to have a **change in the level of care** includes discussing care needs and options with the patient and family to ascertain their feelings and wishes. It also involves discussing changes in the patient's condition and the patient's wishes with the physician. For a patient on palliative care, the change in level of care may involve:

- **Lesser form of care**: This change is indicated because the patient is responding well to treatment, such as may occur following palliative radiotherapy.
- **Hospice care**: If the patient's condition has deteriorated and death is expected within 6 months, then hospice care provides more benefits than palliative care. Patients and family are often unaware of these benefits, so providing information can help them make a decision. Hospice care is appropriate when no further curative treatment is available or when a patient opts to discontinue curative treatments in favor of comfort care.

Pharmacologic Therapies

WHO Pain Ladder

The WHO pain ladder was developed as an algorithm for treating pain through medications with progressively increasing potency. The approach can be used effectively with both adult and pediatric patients. Beginning with the least potent medication option, each step adds a stronger analgesic until optimum pain relief is reached.

The **WHO pain ladder** has three steps.

- **Step 1**: The patient is given a non-opioid medication which may be used alone or in conjunction with other adjuvant therapies.
- **Step 2**: If the patient reports no change in the pain level, mild- to moderate-level pain-relieving opioids are introduced along with adjuvants if they have not been previously introduced.
- **Step 3**: Uncontrolled pain is then treated with opioids for moderate to severe pain. Adjuvants may also be continued.

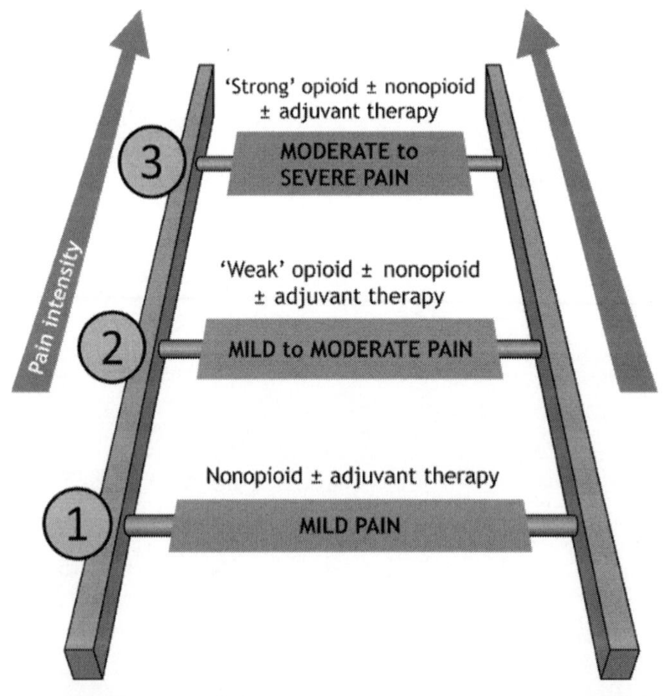

Review Video: Adjuvants
Visit mometrix.com/academy and enter code: 178200

Scheduling of Pain Medications

For mild to moderate pain, patients may take **acetaminophen** alternating with an **NSAID** such as ibuprofen on a regularly scheduled basis or as needed (PRN) at the onset of pain or when pain is anticipated (such as before a dressing change). However, for severe chronic pain, long-acting **opioid pain medications**, such as time-released MS Contin, Duragesic, and OxyContin, should be given regularly around the clock, because these medications help not only control but also prevent pain. The patient should not skip a dose when free of pain, because this makes control more difficult when the pain recurs. In addition to **time-scheduled medications**, the patient may need

short-acting supplementary medications, such as Percocet, to take on a PRN basis. When taking short-acting medications, the patient should take the medication at the onset of pain, before anticipated pain, or at the onset of increased pain, rather than waiting until the pain is severe, because the goal should always be to keep the pain under control.

Acetaminophen

Acetaminophen remains one of the safest analgesics for **long-term use**. It can be used to treat mild pain or as an adjuvant with other analgesics for more severe pain. Nonspecific musculoskeletal pain and osteoarthritis are particularly responsive to acetaminophen therapy. Acetaminophen also has a limited **anti-inflammatory nature**.

Acetaminophen should, however, be used cautiously in persons with altered liver or kidney function, as well as those with a history of significant alcohol use, regardless of liver function compromise. It should be dosed separately from any opioid analgesic, which should be given separately as well. This allows for individual titration of each drug to assess the individual needs and side effects separately.

NSAIDs

NSAIDs act by inhibiting the cyclooxygenase (COX) enzyme, which controls prostaglandin formation. COX-1 affects platelet clumping, gastric blood flow, and mucosal integrity. COX-2 affects pain, inflammation, and fever. COX-1 and 2 inhibitors include aspirin and ibuprofen. Ibuprofen has a lower occurrence of side effects, such as gastric bleeding, than aspirin does. A COX-2 inhibitor, such as Celebrex, must be used with caution due to increased cardiovascular risks when used for over 18 months. NSAIDs are useful for both arthritis and bone cancer pain and work well with opioids for relief of postoperative and other severe pain. NSAIDs may increase the effects of antiseizure drugs and warfarin. Smaller doses are needed if kidney function is impaired.

Review Video: NSAID Side Effects
Visit mometrix.com/academy and enter code: 569064

Local Anesthetic Pain Relief

Local anesthetics block neural conduction of pain through the application of the anesthetic directly to the nerve endings in the area of pain. It can be injected prior to minor surgery or suturing. It can be injected intercostally for thoracic or high abdominal surgeries. The addition of a vasoconstrictor prolongs effectiveness of the anesthetic. A cream containing local anesthetics (EMLA) can be rubbed on the skin to decrease pain from IV starts or lumbar punctures. It should be applied 60-90 minutes prior to the procedure. A lidocaine 5% patch is approved to relieve pain from postherpetic neuralgia. The patient applies up to 3 patches for 12 hours at a time. Local anesthetics can be applied via the use of an epidural catheter to provide pain control for surgery, childbirth, or postoperative pain control. Opioids can be infused along with the anesthetic agent. Patients using an epidural catheter for postoperative pain tend to ambulate sooner, suffer fewer complications as a result, and go home more quickly.

Opioids

Guidelines for Opioid Use

Opioid analgesic therapy is a widely used method of chronic pain control. By adhering to clinical guidelines, pain control can be safely optimized. **Intramuscular administration** should be used as a last resort except in the presence of a "pain emergency" when no other treatment is readily available. Such cases are rare since subcutaneous delivery is almost always an alternative. Noninvasive routes such as **transdermal** and **transmucosal**, which bypass the enteral route, are optimal for continuous pain control and are often effective in eliminating breakthrough pain as well. Changing from one opioid to another, or altering the delivery method, may become necessary under the assumption that incomplete cross-tolerance among opioids occurs. Changing analgesics or method of delivery may result in a decreased drug requirement. When altering opioid delivery regimens, use **morphine equivalents** as the common factor for all dose conversions. This method will help reduce medication errors. Side effects such as sedation, constipation, nausea, and myoclonus should be anticipated in every care plan, and require both prevention and treatment methods.

Side Effects of Opioid Analgesics

Examples of **opioid analgesics** are numerous and include morphine, hydromorphone, oxymorphone, methadone, meperidine, fentanyl, sufentanil, alfentanil, levorphanol, codeine, oxycodone, hydrocodone, propoxyphene, pentazocine, nalbuphine, and buprenorphine. Opioid analgesics have multiple effects on most of the organ systems of the body. Central nervous system (CNS) effects include respiratory depression, analgesia, euphoria, sedation, miosis, cough suppression, truncal rigidity, nausea, and vomiting. Cardiovascular effects are usually slight and include bradycardia, hypotension, reduced blood volume, and increased cerebral blood flow. Gastrointestinal effects can include constipation, decreased gastric motility, and decreased hydrochloric acid. Genitourinary effects are urinary retention and decreased renal function. Other effects are sweating, flushing, and histamine release with itching.

Opioid Use During Last Few Hours of Life

Assessment of pain continues in the **last hours of life**, and medication is adjusted according to assessment. Pain does not necessarily increase as death approaches. It can be assumed that if pain was present prior to loss of consciousness it will continue in the patient's unconscious state. It should be assessed for and treated accordingly. Research has confirmed that administering opioids at the end of life does not hasten nor prolong the dying process. The patient's **prior medication regimen** should be continued. However, adjustments may be made in consideration of reduced renal or hepatic clearance. The **route of administration** should also be assessed for appropriateness and adjusted as needed (e.g., loss of consciousness, inability to swallow).

Oral Transmucosal Fentanyl Citrate

Oral transmucosal fentanyl citrate consists of **fentanyl** on an oral applicator. The patient applies the dosage (starting at 200 mcg) to the **buccal mucosa** between the cheek and gum for rapid absorption and subsequent pain relief. This makes transmucosal fentanyl particularly useful for managing **breakthrough pain**. Pain relief generally begins within 5 minutes, but the patient should be instructed to wait 15 minutes after the previous dose has been completed before taking another dose. Swallowing even part of the dose rather than having it completely absorbed through the oral mucosa can affect the timing of pain relief onset. **Peak effect** occurs in 20-40 minutes with the total pain relief duration lasting 2-3 hours. Side effects can include somnolence, nausea, and dizziness. Consuming drinks such as coffee, tea, and juices that alter the oral secretion pH can also alter the absorption rate of transmucosal fentanyl.

Methadone

Methadone is useful for treating **severe or chronic pain** and may be particularly helpful in the presence of **neuropathic pain**. It has a long-acting pain relief factor for a lower cost than many comparable medications. However, the exact dosing ratios with morphine remain unclear within the available research. Metabolism of methadone can also be swayed (either increased or decreased) by many other medications normally taken by patients with chronic conditions. Methadone can also be used to treat opioid addiction. US law for the prescription of methadone for addiction in detoxification or maintenance programs requires a special license and patient enrollment. The words "for pain" need to be clearly stated in the prescription. Methadone can cause drowsiness, weakness, headache, nausea, vomiting, constipation, sweating, and flushing, as well as sedation, decreased respirations, or an irregular heart rate.

Oxycodone

Oxycodone, a synthetic formulation, is a long-acting opioid for **moderate to severe pain relief**. Side effects are similar to those of morphine. It has a similar pain relief ratio, with the possibility of less nausea and vomiting. Because of its extended-release nature, the medication cannot be cut or crushed for administration. Oxycodone does not carry any greater addiction risk than other types of opioids; however, public sensationalism related to this formulation may create hesitation for use among patients. Pharmacies may also limit the amount of this medication they will make available to an individual. Oxycodone should be used cautiously in patients with a history of hypothyroidism, Addison's disease, urethral stricture, prostatic hypertrophy, or lung or liver disease.

Hydromorphone

Hydromorphone is available as tablets, liquid, suppository, and parenteral formulations. It offers the advantage of being synthetic, allowing for its use in the presence of a true **morphine allergy**. It is also helpful when significant side effects have occurred in the past or pain has been inadequately controlled with other medications. It may also be useful for controlling cough. However, neurotoxicity may occur, particularly myoclonus, hyperalgesia, and seizures. It should also be used cautiously in the presence of kidney, liver, heart, and thyroid disease, seizure disorders, respiratory disease, prostatic hypertrophy, or urinary problems. Common *side effects* include dizziness, lightheadedness, drowsiness, upset stomach if taken without food, vomiting, and constipation.

Titration of Morphine for Pain Control

Morphine titration protocols vary according to the type of morphine used, the severity of pain, and the patient's tolerance:

Type	Peak	Duration (hours)
Short-acting	60 minutes	4-5
Long-acting	3-4 hours	8-24
IM	30-60 minutes	4-5
SQ	50-90 minutes	4-5
IV	20 minutes	4-5
Rectal	20-60 minutes	3-7

For example, **optimal dosage** is usually calculated by starting with short-acting oral morphine at 30 mg every 3-4 hours with doses increased by 25-50% for moderate pain or 50-100% for severe pain each time until the patient has at least 50% reduction in pain on a scale of 1-10 or a behavior scale. The dose may need to be reduced if excessive sedation occurs. Once the patient's pain is controlled on short-acting morphine and 24-hour dosage needs are calculated, the patient could be switched to extended-release. **Breakthrough pain** is usually treated with dosages that are 10% of the 24-hour dose. Dosages may be repeated or increased if there is inadequate relief of pain at the peak time. Increasing the dose prior to peak time will result in increased drowsiness.

Morphine Use for Chronic Cancer Pain

One advantage of morphine for chronic cancer pain is that it has no **ceiling dose**. As tolerance to the medication increases or the disease progresses in severity, the dose can be gradually increased to an infinite level. It is also available in many different forms for administration, including intravenous, intramuscular, immediate release, sustained release, long-acting, liquid oral preparations, and suppositories. Morphine is often used as the **equivalency standard** for other opioid analgesics. Common *side effects* of morphine include sedation, respiratory depression, itching, nausea, chronic spasms or twitching of muscle groups, and constipation. Constipation is experienced by all patients receiving opioids. This inevitability should be planned for and treated aggressively. Hallucinations are common when morphine is initiated. After the first few days, most patients will overcome the respiratory depression, nausea, itching, and extreme sedation as tolerance for the medication is developed.

Dosages for Morphine, Codeine, Hydromorphone, and Levorphanol

The dosages for both the enteral and parenteral routes of morphine, codeine, hydromorphone, and levorphanol are as follows:

- **Morphine**: Enteral dosage is 30 mg (available as continuous and sustained-release formulations to last 12-24 hours); parenteral dosage is 10 mg.
- **Codeine**: Enteral dosage is 200 mg (not generally recommended); parenteral dosage is 130 mg.
- **Hydromorphone**: Enteral dosage is 7.5 mg (available as a continuous-release formula lasting 24 hours); parenteral dosage is 1.5 mg.
- **Levorphanol**: In acute pain episodes, enteral dosage is 4 mg; parenteral dosage is 2 mg. For chronic pain, dosage is equivalent for both enteral and parenteral at 1 mg. Levorphanol has a long half-life, increasing the chances of dosage accumulation over time.

Adhering to the statement "If the gut works, use it," as much as 90 percent of all patients will at least start out able to use oral medications instead of other routes.

Calculation for Converting Medication Regimen Between Two Opioids

Calculate the current 24-hour drug dose, or the total amount given in a 24-hour period. Multiply the current 24-hour dose times the ratio of the 24-hour equivalent dose for the new drug over the 24-hour equivalent of the old drug. This calculation provides the **equivalent 24-hour dose** for the new drug. Divide the new dose amount by the number of doses to be provided during the day. This amount equals the new **target dosage**.

$$\text{current 24 hr dose} \times \frac{\text{new drug 24 hr equiv dose}}{\text{current drug 24 hr equiv dose}} = \text{new 24 hr dose}$$

$$\frac{\text{new 24 hr dose}}{\text{doses per day}} = \text{new target dosage}$$

Ketamine

Ketamine is a dissociative anesthetic that can provide pain relief as an alternate or complement to an opioid. The dissociative quality is an effective way to help the patient separate from the sensation of pain. Ketamine treatment begins with an initial bolus of 0.1 mg/kg IV. If there is no improvement, a second bolus with double the dosage is provided in 5 minutes. This can be repeated as needed. Boluses should be followed by a decrease in the patient's current opioid dose by 50% and an infusion of ketamine. **Infusion dosing** for ketamine is 0.015 mg/kg/min, or about 1 mg/min for a 70 kg person. If IV access cannot be attained, subcutaneous infusion is a possibility with dosing of 0.3-0.5 mg/kg. Consider concurrent treatment with a **benzodiazepine** to prevent hallucinations or frightful dreams and observe for increased secretions, as these are all possible side effects of ketamine. The secretions may be treated with glycopyrrolate, scopolamine, or atropine as needed.

Treating Breakthrough Pain

The three basic types of breakthrough pain, and their treatment measures are as follows:

- **Incident pain**: Pain that can be specifically tied to an activity or event, such as a dressing change or physical therapy. These events can be anticipated and treated with a rapid-onset, short-acting analgesic just prior to the painful event.
- **Spontaneous pain**: This type of pain is unpredictable and cannot be pinpointed to a relationship with any certain time or event. There is no way to anticipate spontaneous pain. In the presence of neuropathic pain, adjuvant therapy may be useful. Otherwise, a rapid-onset, short-acting analgesic is used.
- **End-of-dose failure**: Pain that specifically occurs at the end of a routine analgesic dosing cycle when medication blood levels begin to taper off. Careful evaluation of end-of-dose failure can help prevent it sooner. It may indicate an increased dose tolerance and the need for medication dose alterations.

Treating Neuropathic Pain

Treatment options for neuropathic pain are often different from the methods used to treat other types of pain. The three drug classes most commonly used and proven effective for treating neuropathic pain are **anticonvulsants**, **anesthetics**, and **antidepressants**. Some are given on an as-needed basis, but most require consistent dosing with **24-hour symptom control**. Examples of the most common medications include amitriptyline, nortriptyline, duloxetine, gabapentin, topical lidocaine, opioids, and pregabalin. Medication choice is dependent on factors such as the type and progression of the disorder and the associated physical and emotional problems, such as nerve injury, muscle weakness or spasms, anxiety, depression, or sleep disturbances.

Review Video: Neuropathic Pain
Visit mometrix.com/academy and enter code: 780523

Treating Bone Pain

Treatment options for bone pain may depend on the causative agent related to the pain, such as the primary cancer site, severely weakened bones, or fractures. **Systemic treatment choices** include chemotherapy, radiation, and hormone therapy. **Hormone therapy** is used in the presence of estrogen and androgen receptors within the cancer cells. **Bisphosphonates**, such as ibandronate, zoledronate, and alendronate, may help strengthen the bones, slow damage, and prevent fractures; they can also help reduce pain. However, side effects can include fatigue, fever, nausea, vomiting, and anemia. **Surgery** may also be considered to remove cancerous cells or reinforce weakened areas of bone. **Opioids** and **NSAIDs/COX-2 inhibitors** are most often used for pain relief and need to be provided on a consistent basis.

Morphine combined with ibuprofen provides the benefit of a centrally acting opioid with a peripherally acting NSAID. Ibuprofen also acts as an effective adjuvant analgesic agent to enhance the relief provided by the opioid without increasing opioid side effects.

Measures Taken During Pain Crisis

During a pain crisis, assess for a change in the mechanism or location of the pain and attempt to differentiate between **terminal anxiety** or agitation and the **physical causes** of pain. Begin with a rapid increase in **opioid treatment**. If the pain is unresponsive to opioid titration, switching to

benzodiazepines, such as diazepam and lorazepam, may produce a more effective response. If terminal symptoms remain unresponsive, assess for **drug absorption**. While invasive routes of medication delivery are generally avoided unless necessary, the only guaranteed route of drug delivery is the IV route. If there is any question about absorption, it is appropriate to establish parenteral access. IM delivery should be considered as a last resort. When all accessible resources have been exhausted, seek a pain management consultation as quickly as possible. Alternative methods of terminal pain control include radiotherapy, anesthetic, or neuroablative procedures.

Concerns Surrounding Use of Pain Medications with End-of-Life Patients

Common concerns surrounding the use of pain medications with end-of-life patients include:

- **Adequacy**: Patients are often concerned that medication may not be adequate to control pain and that chronic or breakthrough pain will occur. Patients may be concerned that if they take adequate pain medication, it will be less effective later when pain may be worse.
- **Sedation/addiction**: Some patients and family members are concerned about the risks of addiction, and others may be concerned about the effects of the medication on the patient's cognition, as some patients may become confused, disoriented, or sedated, depending on the medication or dosage.
- **Adverse effects**: Nausea and vomiting may be almost as debilitating to a patient as the pain it is intended to alleviate. Constipation, a common adverse effect, may be very uncomfortable for a patient. Some medications may result in itching and others may cause myoclonus, both of which are uncomfortable for the patient.

Prescribing Controlled Substances to Patients with Advanced Illness and Addiction Challenges

In the presence of **addiction challenges**, it becomes important to choose a **long-acting opioid** that can facilitate around-the-clock dosing and minimize the need for short-term medications used for breakthrough doses. **Short-term medication** use should be very limited or eliminated entirely if possible. Whenever possible, **nondrug adjuvants** such as relaxation techniques, distraction, biofeedback, TNS, and therapeutic communication should be used in place of short-term medications. When short-term medication therapy is needed, a **nonopioid** is best. Limit the amount of medication available to the patient at any given time and monitor for compliance with pill counts and urine toxicology screens as necessary. In some instances, a referral to an addictions specialist is recommended.

Non-Pharmacologic Interventions and Palliative Sedation

Palliative Surgery

Palliative surgery is sometimes carried out to reduce pain and symptoms although in most cases it does not appreciably prolong life. Palliative surgery may be **cancer-directed**, such as palliative nephrectomy with renal cell carcinoma, partial or total gastrectomy for gastric cancer, or endoscopic paranasal debulking for facial metastasis, and aimed at removing cancerous tissue. Decompression of the vertebra (in the case of bony metastases) and arthroplasty of the femur may be carried out to reduce pain and the risk of pathological fractures. Palliative surgery may also be **non-cancer-directed**, which includes procedures that do not remove cancerous tissue, such as palliative colonic splinting and nerve block procedures. Patients may undergo pleurodesis, thoracentesis, thoracotomy, paracentesis, and pericardiocentesis to relieve discomfort. The risks and pain associated with surgical procedures must be balanced against improvement in the quality of life with consideration of the expected length of survival.

Palliative Stents

A stent is a small tube, usually metal or plastic, that is inserted into a duct, vessel, or canal to maintain patency and relieve symptoms associated with cancer that is causing obstruction. These stents are usually placed with microsurgical techniques. **Common stents** include:

- **Pancreatic stents**: These open the bile duct to allow drainage in order to reduce jaundice and associated discomforts, to reduce pain, and to improve digestion.
- **Duodenal stents**: These are placed to maintain patency of the duodenum, which is often obstructed with pancreatic cancer, as an alternative to stomach bypass surgery and/or to relieve nausea and vomiting. Patients may be restricted to soft foods and fluids after the procedure.
- **Liver stents**: These are placed in the bile duct system to allow bile to drain into the small intestine in order to relieve jaundice and symptoms of liver failure.
- **Colonic stents**: These stents are placed to relieve colorectal blockage and relieve symptoms of bowel obstruction.
- **Ureteral stents**: These stents can be used to prevent urinary retention when ureters are obstructed.

Complications of stents may include infection, perforation, hemorrhage, and migration of the stent. Over time, obstruction may recur, especially with malignancies.

Palliative Radiation

Palliative radiation is used to reduce pain and symptoms. Most palliative radiation is done with external beam radiation therapy. **Radiotherapy** uses include:

- **Bone pain**: Radiotherapy may be utilized to reduce tumor mass, such as with multiple myeloma and bony metastasis, and to reduce pain and risk of fractures, with relief often occurring within days of treatment.
- **Pericardial effusions**: Radiotherapy is most effective in reducing effusions with radiosensitive tumors (leukemias, lymphomas).
- **Hemoptysis associated with lung cancer**: Radiotherapy can control hemoptysis in up to 80% of patients with inoperative lung cancer.

- **Spinal cord compression**: Radiotherapy is the primary treatment to relieve compression and reduce symptoms.
- **Brain tumor**: Radiotherapy may reduce the size of the tumor and associated symptoms, such as headaches and nausea.

Radiation does pose some risks of adverse effects that must be considered in relation to quality of life. Depending on the site of radiation, adverse effects may include fatigue, local skin irritation and burns, hair loss, GI upset (nausea, vomiting, dysphagia, diarrhea), dysuria, depressed immune system, and anemia.

Palliative Chemotherapy

Palliative chemotherapy is used primarily to reduce symptoms and pain by decreasing tumor size, which reduces compression of surrounding tissues, and to prolong life when cancer is advanced. Many chemotherapeutic agents are available, and adverse effects associated with use vary widely but can include nausea and vomiting, anorexia, hair loss, weakness, fatigue, and impaired immune system. **Palliative chemotherapy** is often given in conjunction with palliative radiation. Patients should be well-informed before deciding on a course of palliative chemotherapy and should understand how many cycles will be needed (usually 2 full cycles are given before deciding whether the treatment is effective), how long the cycles will be, what type of adverse effects to expect, what reduction in symptoms is anticipated, and how long studies show that the treatment prolongs life. If the prolongation of life and symptom relief is minimal, the trade-off for decreased quality of life must be considered.

Palliative Sedation

Palliative sedation differs from physician-assisted suicide in that it is primarily intended to provide comfort and alleviate suffering, and the hastening of death that may occur is a secondary effect while the primary purpose of physician-assisted suicide is to bring about a patient's death (even though it is also intended to provide comfort and alleviate suffering). These are legal distinctions. In most states, physician-assisted suicide is illegal, but the US Supreme Court has upheld the rights of individuals to have **palliative sedation** to alleviate symptoms. Midazolam (Versed) 0.5-6.0 mg/hr intravenously is often used for palliative sedation for patients who are highly agitated and in severe uncontrolled pain. Midazolam is a very short-acting benzodiazepine with action beginning within 5 minutes and peaking at 20-60 minutes. Propofol, another IV agent, is also used, with starting doses of 0.25 mg/kg/hr. Palliative sedation is indicated for patients when other medications and therapies have been unable to control their refractory symptoms, such as intractable pain, severe nausea and vomiting, feeling of suffocation, and seizures.

Counseling, Psychological Therapy, and Cognitive Behavioral Therapy

Both patients and their families may benefit from **counseling and psychological therapy**, which may allow them to express feelings and concerns that might otherwise remain hidden. Counseling may help patients/families come to terms with death, dying, and limitations and changes brought about by illness. Grief and bereavement counseling is especially helpful for family members after a patient has died. Pastoral counseling, often carried out by chaplains, pastors, and priests, may facilitate spiritual assessment and provide spiritual support. Psychological therapy may help to treat depression brought about by illness, and specific psychological techniques, such as visualization, relaxation exercises, and cognitive behavioral therapy, may help patients better control pain and reduce stress and anxiety.

Cognitive-behavioral therapy (CBT) focuses on the impact that thoughts have on behavior and feelings and encourages the individual to use the power of rational thought to alter perceptions and behavior. Individuals are assigned "homework" during the sessions to practice new ways of thinking and to develop new coping strategies. The therapist helps the individual identify goals and find ways to achieve them.

Cancer Diets

Cancer diets have been developed based on the premise that some foods "feed" cancer and others kill cancer cells although evidence-based support that the diets alter outcomes is lacking. Some people pursue diet therapy in place of traditional treatments while others use the diet in addition to other treatments. Many utilize a primarily vegan (plant-based) diet, which is usually lacking in vitamin B_{12}. While diets differ somewhat, basic concepts include:

- Avoiding refined carbohydrates (sugar, white flour) and milk products
- Avoiding fatty acids, fried foods, fast foods, and processed foods
- Avoiding alcohol, caffeine, nicotine, and chemicals
- Avoiding meats, such as beef and poultry (purported to interfere with the immune system)
- Avoiding cooking/overcooking and pasteurization (purported to destroy nutrients)
- Utilizing organic fruits and vegetables in order to avoid ingestion of pesticides
- Encouraging raw fruits, raw vegetables, seeds, whole grains, and nuts

Complementary and Alternative Interventions

Complementary Therapy

Complementary therapies are often used, either alone or in conjunction with conventional medical treatment. These methods should be included if this is what the patient/family chooses, empowering the family to take control of their plan of care. Complementary therapies vary widely and most can easily be incorporated. The **National Center for Complementary and Alternative Medicine** recognizes the following:

- **Whole medical systems**: Chinese medicine (acupressure, acupuncture), naturopathic and homeopathic medicines, and Ayurveda
- **Mind-body medicine**: Prayer, artistic creation, music and dance therapy, biofeedback, focused relaxation, and visualization
- **Biological medicine**: Aromatherapy, herbs, plants, trees, vitamins and minerals, and dietary supplements
- **Manipulation**: Massage and spinal manipulation
- **Energy medicines**: Magnets, electric current, pulsed fields, Reiki, qi gong, and laying-on of the hands

Precautions

The use of alternative and complementary therapies should be thoroughly discussed by patients and their physician. Patients should be encouraged to use therapies that are shown to have a beneficial, complementary effect on conventional medical treatment. These therapies include the use of massage, superficial stimulation, relaxation, distraction, hypnosis, and guided imagery.

- Encourage patients to practice the techniques until they are proficient in their use to give them a chance to prove their value.
- Teach the patient how the therapies work to encourage the patient to believe in them to contribute to the placebo effect.
- Caution the patient against abandoning current medical treatment.
- Inform the patient of the high cost of alternate therapies that can divert needed funds and result in little or no benefit.
- Provide the patient with resources in the form of books, pamphlets, and informative websites that prove the results of scientific research so that they can evaluate alternative therapies for themselves.

Whole Medical Systems

Whole medical systems are different philosophies and methods of explaining and treating health and illness. Some systems include:

- **Homeopathic medicine**: This European system uses small amounts of diluted herbs and supplements to help the body to recover from disease by stimulating an immune response.
- **Naturopathic medicine**: This is a European system that uses various natural means (herbs, massage, acupuncture) to support the natural healing forces of the body.
- **Chinese medicine**: Centers on restoring the proper flow of life forces within the body to cure disease by using herbs, acupressure and acupuncture, and meditation.
- **Ayurveda**: This is an Indian system that tries to bring the spirit into harmony with the mind and body to treat disease via yoga, herbs, and massage.

Essential Oils and Cupping

Essential oils (concentrated oils from plants) are either inhaled (aromatherapy) or diluted and applied to the skin. Essential oils are believed to reduce stress, aid sleep, improve dermatitis, and aid digestion. Commonly used essential oils include eucalyptus, lavender, lemon, peppermint, rosemary, rose, and tea tree. Oils may cause skin irritation when applied to the skin.

Cupping is an ancient practice still used in Southeast Asia and the Middle East to reduce pain, promote healing, and improve circulation. With dry cupping, cups are heated by placing something flammable (such as paper or herbs) inside the cup and setting it on fire to heat the cup, which is then immediately placed on the back along the meridians (generally on both sides of the spine) to form a vacuum that draws blood to the skin and causes circular bruises believed to heal that part of the body. Wet cupping includes leaving the heated cup in place for three minutes, removing it, making small cuts in the skin, and then applying suction cups again to withdraw blood. Cupping should be avoided in children under 4 and limited to short periods in older children.

Acupuncture

Alternative systems of medical practice include acupuncture, homeopathy, and naturopathy. **Acupuncture**, an ancient Oriental practice, uses stainless steel or copper needles inserted into superficial skin layers at points where energy or life force called *qi* is believed to occur. The needles are supposed to restore balance and the flow of *qi*. The NIH has recognized the effectiveness of acupuncture for certain side effects of other cancer treatments, such as nausea, vomiting, and pain. However, there is no documented scientific evidence to support the principles expounded. Acupuncturists are certified through either formal coursework or apprenticeships, and there is also board certification in this area for physicians. The needles used are classified as class II, which means they have manufacturing and labeling requirements.

Herbal Remedies and Regulations

In the United States, most **herbal preparations** are classified as dietary supplements. That means that they are not subject to the same rigorous manufacturing, safety, efficacy, and control practices as pharmaceutical drugs. Herbal supplements are only governed by the Dietary Supplement and Health Education Act (DSHEA). As long as no specific disease treatment or curative claims are made, the supplement can be marketed without limitation and safety concerns must be pursued by the FDA after the fact. Nevertheless, some herbal remedies have been undergoing clinical trials in the US to substantiate their health-enhancing or traditional/historical or international use claims. However, the focal point of these studies is still only on the effectiveness of the specific supplement. In Europe, there has been some movement toward greater regulation and licensing of herbal products, but not to the extent of formal drug regulations.

Toxicities Associated with Herbal Remedies

Use of herbal preparations has been associated with a variety of **toxicities**, primarily in categories such as cardiovascular problems, hypersensitivity reactions, disorientation, gastrointestinal problems, and liver malfunction. Because quality control measures are relatively lax for these remedies, contamination from infectious agents and toxic metals can potentially cause other side effects. Many of these herbal medicines **interact with conventional drugs**, thus altering their pharmacodynamics. For example, St. John's wort, which is primarily used for depressive disorders or as a sedative, interacts with a wide range of traditional pharmacologic agents and suppresses their levels in the bloodstream. Kava kava, made from dried roots of a type of pepper bush, is used as a sedative, but it also has been associated with hepatic failure and via interactions with several other drugs can actually induce a comatose state. Ginseng is an Asian remedy touted for its curative properties in a number of diseases. However, it can react with steroidal drugs and induce shaking and manic episodes. These are just a few examples of potential dangers.

Non-Pharmaceutical Pain Relief

Non-pharmaceutical methods to relieve pain that can be used exclusively or combined with medications include massage, heat, cold, electrical stimulation, distraction, relaxation, imagery, visualization, and music. Other **alternatives or adjuncts to pain medication** include hypnosis, magnets, acupuncture, acupressure, and therapeutic touch. Herbs, aromatherapy, reflexology, homeopathic medicine, and prayer may also be accepted by the patient. Any method that the patient feels may help that isn't harmful should be used to help get relief.

Mind-Body Medicine for Pain and Disease

Mind-body medicine (prayer, artistic creation, music and dance, biofeedback, relaxation, and visualization) can help distract people from pain or other symptoms if they are able to concentrate on the method. This can result in the transfer of less painful stimuli to the brain by stimulating the **descending control system**. These methods work if the patient can use them to create alternate sensations in the brain, but will not work if the patient is unable to concentrate due to intense pain.

Relaxation that occurs as a result of using these methods helps to reduce muscular tension that can make pain worse and reduces fatigue caused by chronic pain. Relaxation has been proven to be the most helpful after surgery. Postoperative patients report a greater feeling of control over their pain and tend to request fewer opioids to control pain. Biofeedback can help patients to recognize the feelings of both tension and relaxation and provide a way to indicate their success in managing muscle tension.

Use of Visualization

There are a number of methods used for **visualization** to reduce anxiety and promote healing. Some include audiotapes with guided imagery, such as self-hypnosis tapes, but the patient can be taught basic **techniques** that include:

- Sit or lie comfortably in a **quiet place** away from distractions.
- Concentrate on **breathing** while taking long slow breaths.
- **Close the eyes** to shut out distractions and create an image in the mind of the place or situation desired.
- Concentrate on that **image**, engaging as many senses as possible and imaging details.
- If the mind wanders, breathe deeply and **bring consciousness back** to the image or concentrate on breathing for a few moments and then return to the imagery.
- End with positive imagery.

Sometimes, patients are resistive at first or have a hard time maintaining focus, so **guiding** them through visualization for the first few times can be helpful.

Stimulation of the Skin to Reduce Pain

Skin, muscles, fascia, tendons, and the cornea contain **nociceptors** that are nerve endings that respond to painful stimuli. Massage, transcutaneous electrical nerve stimulation (TENS), heat and cold provide stimulation to other nerves that transfer only sensation, not pain. These signals block some of the transfer of the nociceptor impulses:

- **Massage** not only sends alternate sensation to the brain, but also results in relaxation that decreases the muscular tension that contributes to pain.
- **TENS** works well on incisional and neuromuscular pain by providing a gentle electrical stimulation that overrides the painful impulses from the area and may stimulate endorphins.
- **Heat therapy** increases blood flow and oxygen to promote healing and stimulates neural receptors, decreasing pain. Heat also helps loosen tense muscles that may be contributing to pain.
- **Cold therapy** decreases circulation and reduces production of chemicals related to inflammation, thereby reducing pain.

Temperature-Controlled Therapies

Methods of Heating and Cooling

There are a number of different ways to **heat** (thermotherapy) or **cool** (cryotherapy) for **healing**:

- **Conduction**: Conveyance of heat, cold, or electricity through direct contact with the skin, such as with hot baths, ice packs, and electrical stimulation.
- **Convection**: Indirect transmission of heat in a liquid or gas by circulation of heated particles, such as with whirlpools and paraffin soaks.
- **Conversion**: Heating that results from converting a form of energy into heat, such as with diathermy and ultrasound.
- **Evaporation**: Cooling caused by liquids that evaporate into gases on the skin with a resultant cooling effect, such as with perspiration or vapo-coolant sprays.
- **Radiation**: Heating that results from transfer of heat through light waves or rays, such as with infrared or ultraviolet light.

Superficial Heat

Superficial heat with externally applied heat sources penetrates only the superficial layers of the skin (1-2 cm after about 30 minutes), but it is believed to relax deeper muscles by reflex, decrease pain, and increase metabolisms (2-3 times for every 10 °C increase in skin temperature). Therapeutic temperature range is 40-45 °C. **Superficial heat modalities** include:

- **Moist heat packs** placed on the skin and secured by several layers of towels to provide insulation, applied for 15-30 minutes.
- **Paraffin baths** (52-54 °C) with the hand, foot, or elbow dipped 7 times, cooling between dippings, and then wrapping with plastic and towels for 20 minutes.
- **Fluidotherapy** uses hot-air warmed (38.8-47.8 °C) cellulose particles into which a hand or foot is submerged for 20-30 minutes.

Passive and active range of motion exercises are done after superficial heat treatment. Contraindications include cardiac disease, peripheral vascular disease, malignant tumor, bleeding, and acute inflammation.

Deep heat differs from superficial heat in that the heat is generated internally using ultrasound, short wave, and microwave diathermy rather than applied to the surface of the skin. Deep heating has penetrance to 3-5 cm.

Therapeutic Ultrasound

Ultrasound treats soft-tissue injuries (such as myositis, bursitis, and tendinitis) with sound waves (frequency 0.8-3 MHz). Ultrasound utilizes a **piezoelectric crystal** that vibrates, producing sound waveforms, which are transmitted from the transducer through a gel substance into the tissue. The sound waves bounce off of the bone in an irregular pattern that causes an increase in temperature in the connective tissue, such as collagen fibers. Temperatures of the tissue may increase up to 43.5 °C, increasing metabolism in the area, neural conduction, as well as blood flow. Ultrasound is used to **decrease both contractures and scarring**. During treatment, the transducer passes in a circular motion about the skin surface, staying in contact with the gel medium. If a distal limb is submerged in water, the treatment is given with the head of the transducer 0.5-1.0 in from the skin surface. Treatment is followed by range of motion exercises, passive and active. Contraindications are similar to other heat-producing modalities and include peripheral vascular disease, but ultrasound may be used over metal prostheses.

TENS

Transcutaneous electrical nerve stimulation (TENS) uses electrical stimulation to stimulate **peripheral sensory nerve fibers** to reduce acute or recurrent pain. TENS machines may be 2-lead or 4-lead and have adjustments for both frequency (1-20 Hz) and pulse width (50-300 µs, 10-50 mA). Stimulation can be intermittent or continuous. TENS units are small and battery-powered with wires and adhesive electrodes attached so that they can be worn while the person goes about usual activities. The positioning of the electrodes and the settings depend upon the site and type of injury, following guidelines provided by the manufacturer. The TENS machine can be used for a number of hours, but if used for days at a time, it will be less effective. TENS treatment is contraindicated with demand pacemakers and should not be used on the head or neck or over irritated skin.

Hospice and Palliative Care Emergencies

Autonomic Dysreflexia

Autonomic dysreflexia can occur with central cord lesions at or above T6 and can result in encephalopathy and shock if undiagnosed and untreated. Autonomic dysreflexia occurs after the initial spinal shock has resolved. Onset is often very sudden and constitutes a medical emergency. Common causes include distended bladder, fecal impaction, pressure sores, tight clothing, hyperthermia, and other painful stimuli.

Symptoms
- Hypertension, severe pounding headache, increased ICP, and/or rupture of cerebral vessel
- Bradycardia, other cardiac arrhythmias
- Diaphoresis, piloerection, flushing of skin below level of injury and pallor above
- Nasal congestion
- Blurred vision, spots in visual field
- Seizures

Treatment
- Elevate head immediately to reduce blood pressure.
- Identify and rectify cause (check bladder, bowels, skin, clothing, temperature).
- If related to bladder distention, catheterize and drain the bladder slowly.
- If initial treatment is not successful in reversing symptoms, then give medications (IV antihypertensives, such as hydralazine, and antispasmodics).

Seizures

Common causes of seizures at the end-of-life include brain tumors, medications (TCAs, phenothiazines, butyrophenones, opioids), and infection. In hospice and palliative care patients, the most common types of **seizures** include:

- **Simple partial (focal)**: Unilateral motor symptoms including somatosensory, psychic, and autonomic
- **Aversive**: Eyes and head turned away from focal side
- **Sylvan (usually during sleep)**: Tonic-clonic movements of the face, salivation, and arrested speech
- **Tonic-clonic (general)**: Occurs without warning
  - Tonic period (10-30 seconds): Eyes roll upward with loss of consciousness, arms flexed, stiffen in symmetric tonic contraction of body, apneic with cyanosis and salivating.
  - Clonic period (up to 30 minutes, but usually ~30 seconds). Violent rhythmic jerking with contraction and relaxation. May be incontinent of urine and feces. Contractions slow and then stop.

During a seizure, the patient should be unrestrained but positioned on the side to prevent aspiration. Anticonvulsants or other drugs (phenytoin, carbamazepine, phenobarbital, valproic acid, divalproex, midazolam) may be administered to prevent or control seizures. The seizure should be timed, and the patient protected from harm.

Hemorrhage

Hemorrhage may be internal (hemorrhagic stroke, GI bleeding) or external (bleeding wound, tumor) and may be associated with disease (leukemia, disseminated intravascular coagulopathy, AIDS, uremia), clotting disorders (thrombocytopenia), tumor necrosis (eroded vessels), trauma (penetrating injuries), and medications (warfarin, NSAIDs, beta-lactam antibiotics, aspirin). Symptoms (pallor, hypotension, tachycardia) are usually evident with acute rapid hemorrhage when about 20% of blood volume is lost because the body is not able to compensate for the loss. Hemorrhage may be treated aggressively or palliatively, depending on the patient's condition and advance directive and the site/extent of bleeding, but steps are generally taken to **control bleeding**:

- Apply pressure dressing to control external bleeding.
- Provide fluid resuscitation.
- Stop anticoagulant drugs and administer reversal agents.
- Treat coagulopathy.
- Carry out invasive interventions: surgery, radiotherapy, embolization, endoscopic procedures (balloon tamponade, lavage), and cryosurgery.
- Apply hemostatic agents, dressings.
- PPIs and H2 receptor antagonists (gastric bleeding).
- Administer tranexamic acid.
- Administer blood products, such as packed red blood cells.

SVCS

Superior vena cava syndrome (SVCS) is the result of a **partial occlusion of the superior vena cava**, which results in decreased venous blood flow from the head and neck to the right atrium. The blockage may result from cancerous growths. This is considered an emergency condition marked by headache, facial edema, hoarseness, dyspnea, and swollen arms. In situations of rapid onset, the loss of circulation can be life threatening. The severity and timing of symptom onset can be gradual or acute. Patients may report subtle signs such as swelling in the morning hours, or increasing discomfort with bending forward or stooping. The most common complaint is dyspnea. Other physical findings can include vein distention in the neck and chest, a ruddy complexion or cyanosis, tachypnea, stridor, orthopnea, hoarseness, nasal stuffiness, periorbital and conjunctivae edema. As symptoms progress, cerebral edema will occur, potentially leading to stupor, coma, seizures, or death.

Life Support Devices

Discontinuing Life Support

Discontinuation or withholding of life support often occurs when a patient is dying and unlikely to benefit from treatment. Patients (and surrogates if the patient is unable to make decisions) have the right to refuse life-supporting/life-prolonging therapy. Before withdrawing life-support, a DNR order should be documented as well as the reason and rationale for discontinuation of treatment. Most commonly, life-supporting therapies are withdrawn in the following sequence:

1. Blood products, such as packed red blood cells
2. Hemodialysis
3. Vasopressors
4. Mechanical ventilation
5. Total parenteral nutrition
6. Antibiotics (allowing infection to take its course)
7. Intravenous fluids
8. Tube feedings

Bedside monitors should be shut off during the withdrawal procedures. The family should be included in decision-making and apprised of the steps taken to discontinue life support and to provide for the patient's comfort. The time to death after discontinuation of treatment varies depending on a number of factors, but discontinuation of ventilation usually results in death within a few minutes or hours while discontinuation of hemodialysis usually results in death in 2-3 days.

Removal of Mechanical Ventilation

Steps for the removal of mechanical ventilation include:

1. Decrease provided analgesia (opioid) and decrease intermittent mandatory ventilation to <10, then discontinue neuromuscular blockade so that the level of discomfort can be more accurately assessed.
2. Turn off alarms and monitors.
3. Position patient at 30° or higher and suction mouth if secretions are copious.
4. Set PEEP to 0.
5. Gradually reduce the fractional oxygen content (FiO_2).
6. Reduce or stop mandatory inspirations.
7. Reduce level of pressure support.
8. Place T-piece to flow-by.
9. Extubate.
10. Administer humidified oxygen.
11. Administer opioid (morphine, fentanyl, or midazolam) and/or diazepam if the patient exhibits signs of distress.

The time period from beginning of the weaning process to extubation usually takes 15-60 minutes.

Discontinuing Nutrition and Hydration

Artificial nutrition and hydration (per TPN, tube feedings, IV fluids) are medical treatments and can be withdrawn along with other treatments for patients who are nearing death or in a permanent vegetative state. As the patient's systems begin to shut down, continuing artificial nutrition and hydration can increase edema, secretions, and heart failure, resulting in increased discomfort. Additionally, TPN and tube feedings may lead to a number of different complications. As patients near death, they typically do not experience hunger or thirst. Some healthcare providers feel that providing fluids to dying patients may be a comfort measure, but most adverse effects (dry mouth, cracked lips) can be alleviated effectively with good medical and nursing care. Often the decision regarding artificial hydration rests with the patient or family, but if hydration is continued, a minimal volume should be used to avoid fluid overload.

Turning Off LVAD and ICD

Ventricular assist devices (VAD) can provide support to the left (most common; LVAD) or right ventricle or both. With most devices, blood drains from the base of the left ventricle into the pump through an inflow cannula and back into the aorta through an outflow cannula. The LVAD pump is placed preperitoneally in the abdomen with electrical cables and air vent tunneled through a percutaneous line to the external controller and battery pack. The **implantable cardioverter defibrillator (ICD)** is usually placed in the upper chest with electrodes into the right atrium. It paces the heart and delivers a shock when necessary. Before the devices are discontinued, the patient is usually sedated to reduce the perception of dyspnea associated with abrupt reduction in cardiac output, especially with the LVAD. In most cases, patients will die within minutes of the LVAD being shut off, but if the patient has some residual cardiac function, death may be delayed for a few days. Death after removal of the ICD may vary depending on residual cardiac function.

Withholding or Withdrawing Medications from Dying Patients

Withholding or withdrawing medications of dying patients must include the following considerations:

- Antihypertensives and other drugs (diuretics, antibiotics, hormones, antidysrhythmics, hypoglycemic agents, and laxatives) that do not directly contribute to patient comfort are usually discontinued in the final days.
- Abrupt discontinuation of corticosteroids can cause severe effects, so discontinuation should be tapered. If used to reduce cerebral edema and intracranial pressure in order to control pain and seizures, as the corticosteroid dose is tapered, the dosage of anticonvulsant should be increased.
- Medications that are usually continued as long as possible include sedatives and analgesics and medications to control symptoms, such as antipyretics, antiemetics, anticholinergics, and anticonvulsants.
- Oral medications can be continued as long as a patient can swallow, often in liquid form rather than pills or capsules. Other medications may be administered parenterally.
- Patients should be medicated prior to extubation, and additional medications should be available to control symptoms. The medications that are most indicated to relieve a sense of breathlessness are opioids. Benzodiazepines are also usually administered to relieve anxiety. Oxygen is usually continued at about 21%.

Education and Communication

Age-Appropriate Teaching Methods

Bandura's Theory of Social Learning

In the 1970s, Bandura proposed the theory of social learning, in which he posited that learning develops from observing, organizing, and rehearsing behavior that has been modeled. Bandura believed that people are more likely to adopt the behavior if they value the outcomes, if the outcomes have functional value, and if the person modeling the behavior is similar to the learner and is admired because of status. Behavior is the result of observation of behavioral, environmental, and cognitive interactions. There are **four conditions** required for modeling:

- **Attention**: The degree of attention paid to modeling can depend on many variables (physical, social, and environmental).
- **Retention**: People's ability to retain models depends on symbolic coding, creating mental images, organizing thoughts, and rehearsing (mentally or physically).
- **Reproduction**: The ability to reproduce a model depends on physical and mental capabilities.
- **Motivation**: Motivation may derive from past performances, rewards, or vicarious modeling.

Transtheoretical Model of Change

The transtheoretical model of change puts forth concepts applicable to the process of educating patients and their family members. The **stages** of the transtheoretical model of change include the following:

1. The first stage is **precontemplation**. At this point, the patient is not aware of any need for a change in the health behavior.
2. In the next stage, **contemplation**, the patient begins to realize why the change may be necessary after recognizing that the health behavior in question is unhealthy and weighing the consequences of continuing this behavior.
3. During the stage of **preparation**, the patient imagines making the change at a future time and starts to formulate a plan to do so.
4. The **action** stage occurs when the patient makes specific modifications in health behavior and begins to note the resulting positive changes.
5. During the **maintenance** stage, the patient is able to implement the change over time by utilizing strategies to prevent a return to previously unhealthy behaviors.
6. **Termination** is the stage at which a patient has incorporated the changed behavior into daily functioning, and the patient will not resume the previous unhealthy behavior.

Kurt Lewin

Force Field Analysis

Force field analysis was designed by Kurt Lewin, a social psychologist, to analyze both the driving forces and the restraining forces for change:

- **Driving forces** instigate and promote change, such as leaders, incentives, and competition.
- **Restraining forces** resist change, such as poor attitudes, hostility, inadequate equipment, or insufficient funds.

The educator can use this force field analysis diagram to discuss variables related to a proposed change in process:

- Write the proposed change in the center column.
- Brainstorm and list driving forces and opposed restraining forces. Score the forces. (When driving and restraining forces are in balance, this is a state of equilibrium or the status quo.)
- Discuss the value of the proposed change.
- Develop a plan to diminish or eliminate restraining forces.

Lewin's Model of Change Theory

Lewin's model of change theory may be used to help some patients make decisions for change. Patients can be educated about the need for change and can be assisted with making alterations in behavior or thoughts in order to better facilitate change; however, only the patient can truly implement the change permanently. Lewin's concept of change theory involves a three-part process:

- **Unfreezing** is the part of the model in which the patient becomes open to change, sees a need for it, and removes the boundaries inhibiting change.
- The patient then makes the **actual change** according to expected outcomes and goals.
- Finally, **refreezing** is the process of maintaining the change so that it becomes a habit, and one that the patient is likely to uphold for a long period of time.

Lewin's theory also involves either driving forces or restraining forces. Driving forces are those outside measures that support the change, while restraining forces inhibit success in implementing the change.

Learning Styles

Not all patients are aware of their preferred learning style. A range of teaching materials/methods that are age appropriate and relate to all three learning preferences—visual, auditory, kinesthetic—should be available. Part of assessment for teaching involves choosing the right approach based on observation and feedback. Often presenting learners with different options gives a clue to their preferred learning style. Some individuals have a combined learning style:

Visual learners	**Learn best by seeing and reading**: Provide written directions, picture guides, or demonstrate procedures. Use charts and diagrams. Provide photos and videos.
Auditory learners	**Learn best by listening and talking**: Explain procedures while demonstrating and have the learner repeat. Plan extra time to discuss and answer questions. Provide audiotapes.
Kinesthetic learners	**Learn best by handling, doing, and practicing**: Provide hands-on experience throughout teaching. Encourage handling of supplies/equipment. Allow the learner to demonstrate. Minimize instructions and allow the person to explore equipment and procedures.

Learning Principles

Young Adulthood

Young adulthood encompasses the ages of 20-40 during which people are usually in the cognitive stage of formal operations and psychological stage of intimacy vs. isolation. **Young adults** tend to be autonomous and self-directed and have intrinsic motivation to learn. Their personal experience may enhance or interfere with their learning. Young adults tend to be competency-based leaners who are able to make decisions and analyze critically. The provider should assess learner motivation and try to identify obstacles to learning and support systems. Teaching strategies include:

- Utilize problem-centered learning.
- Allow people to learn at their own paces and draw on experiential learning.
- Encourage people to participate actively.
- Utilize roleplaying, hands-on practice, and immediate application.
- Keep materials and presentations well organized and clear.
- Recognize the social roles of learners.
- Encourage self-directed learning.
- Focus on health promotion.

Middle-Aged Adulthood

Middle-aged adulthood encompasses the ages of 41-64 during which people are in the cognitive stage of formal operations and the psychological stage of generativity vs stagnation. **Middle-aged adults** tend to be at the peak of their careers with a well-developed sense of self although they may have concerns about physical changes. They may explore alternative lifestyles, question achievements, and reexamine values and goals. They may desire change but still have confidence in their abilities. The provider should assess learner motivation and try to identify obstacles to learning and support systems. Teaching strategies include:

- Be flexible but organized and efficient.
- Assess and recognize potential technology gaps.
- Encourage people to utilize experiential learning.
- Review study skills.
- Relate learning to life concerns.
- Provide reassurance and positive reinforcement.
- Modify approaches for physical disabilities or impairments.

Older Adulthood

Older adulthood is age 65 and older, during which the person is in the cognitive stage of formal operations and the psychological stage of ego integrity vs. despair. The provider should encourage participation from **older adults**, assess coping mechanisms, and provide supplementary materials to reinforce learning. Teaching strategies include:

- Spend a little time getting to know the person so the person is more relaxed and receptive to learning.
- Determine what information is critical and what is non-essential.
- Evaluate the person's learning style and previous knowledge about the topic.
- Plan ample time for each session of instruction.
- Ensure that sessions are closely spaced to reinforce learning.
- Provide the person ample time to practice.

- Allow the person to guide the pace of the session as much as possible and encourage feedback.
- Prepare age-appropriate handouts at an accessible reading level with large-size font.
- Provide materials (pencil, paper) in case the patient wants to make notes.
- Be supportive, patient, and enthusiastic.

Therapeutic Environment Conducive to Learning

Factors to consider when establishing a therapeutic environment conducive to learning include:

- **Temperature**: The temperature should be comfortable for the patient. If the room temperature cannot be adjusted, then a fan or extra blankets may be used to ensure patient comfort.
- **Lighting**: The lighting should be at an adequate level to view materials but should not be glaring or excessively bright.
- **Noise**: The environment should be as free of extraneous noise as possible. A quiet space is ideal, but if that's not possible, the door to the room should be closed.
- **Comfort**: The patient should receive adequate analgesia because pain is very distracting. Additionally, the patient and family should be in positions of comfort. For example, the patient may be most comfortable sitting in bed or in a comfortable chair.
- **Timing**: The provider should discuss the best time with the patient and family. If the patient has pain, then learning is usually optimal during the time the pain is best controlled. Patients should exhibit readiness to learn.

Characteristics of Formal Education

Formal education is planned and developed to meet particular needs, such as educating patients about pain control and the use of a PCA. Planning includes carrying out a needs assessment and then developing a syllabus and materials in support of the topics that is appropriate for the students. Characteristics common to **formal education** include:

- **Setting**: Formal education usually takes place in a classroom or specified area.
- **Timing**: Classes are scheduled on specific dates and times.
- **Structure**: An instructor presents material and leads the class. The instructor should be credentialed, certified, or qualified to teach the material.
- **Materials**: May include overhead projection, equipment, books, pamphlets, handouts, videos, and audio recordings.
- **Assessment**: Some type of assessment is normally included, such as a test or a return demonstration.
- **Class size**: While formal education is usually directed at a group, the size may vary, and in some cases a formal education module may be utilized for individuals.

Characteristics of Informal Education

Informal education takes place outside of the classroom and is generally unplanned and follows no particular format. Informal education most often occurs in the course of conversation with a patient and family members. While informal education is not planned in the same way as formal education, being knowledgeable and educated about disease and patient concerns prepares the nurse when opportunities for informal education occur. Characteristics of **informal education** include:

- **Setting**: Informal education can take place anywhere.
- **Timing**: It often happens as an immediate response to patient's questions and needs and to observations.

- **Structure**: Patient or family and instructor (nurse) have a reciprocal exchange.
- **Materials**: Usually those on hand, such as equipment being used during the exchange, although the nurse may offer to provide additional materials.
- **Assessment**: The nurse can assess through informal questioning: "Did you understand?" or "Do you have any more questions?"
- **Class size**: Informal education almost always happens as one-on-one exchanges although in some cases family members or others may be present and participate.

Readiness to Learn

Learner characteristics related to readiness to learn should be assessed because if people are not ready, instruction is of little value. Often readiness is indicated when people ask questions or show interest in procedures. There are a number of factors related to **readiness to learn**:

- **Physical factors**: There are a number of physical factors than can affect ability. Manual dexterity may be required to complete a task, and this varies by age and condition. Hearing or vision deficits may impact ability. Complex tasks may be too difficult for some because of weakness or cognitive impairment, and modifications of the environment may be needed. Health status, age, and gender may all impact the ability to learn.
- **Experience with learning**: People's experience with learning can vary widely and is affected by their ability to cope with changes, their personal goals, motivation to learn, and cultural background. People may have widely divergent ideas about what constitutes illness and treatment. Lack of English skills may make learning difficult and prevent people from asking questions.
- **Mental/emotional status**: The support system and motivation may impact readiness. Anxiety, fear, or depression about the condition can make learning very difficult because people cannot focus on learning, so the nurse must spend time to reassure them and wait until they are emotionally more receptive.
- **Knowledge/education**: The knowledge base of patients, their cognitive abilities, and their learning styles all affect their readiness to learn. The nurse should always begin by assessing what knowledge the people already have about their disease, condition, or treatment and then build from that base. People with little medical experience may lack knowledge of basic medical terminology, interfering with their ability and readiness to learn.

Selection of Teaching Methods

There are many teaching methods, and the nurse must prepare, present, and coordinate a wide range of educational workshops, lectures, discussions, and one-on-one instructions on any chosen topic. All types of classes may be needed, depending upon the purpose and material:

- **Educational workshops** are usually conducted with small groups, allowing for maximal participation. They are especially good for demonstrations and practice sessions.
- **Lectures** are often used for more academic or detailed information that may include questions and answers but limits discussion. An effective lecture should include some audiovisual support.
- **Discussions** are best with small groups so that people can actively participate. This is good for problem solving exercises.
- **One-on-one instruction** is especially helpful for targeted instruction in procedures for individuals or for those who need additional assistance.
- **Computer/internet modules** are good for independent learners but may be valuable supplements to traditional classroom presentations, especially if they are interactive.

Teaching Tools Available for Patient Education

Teaching tools include:

- **Print materials**: Print materials may be provided before, during, or after class and can include books, journals, and copies of articles, handouts, reference cards, and posters.
- **Electronics/audio-visual**: Computer-assisted learning modules, tablet applications, and podcasts are especially valuable for independent study. Videos and audio-recordings may be used independently or to supplement a class presentation. For example, videos may be used for demonstrations if equipment is not available or to show how to use equipment.
- **Display**: Various types of displays can be used, including whiteboards, electronic whiteboards, flipcharts, and slide show presentations.
- **Internet resources**: Databases, NIH/CDC sites, Medline can provide excellent reference materials. Government sites often offer brochures and pamphlets for free download.
- **Equipment**: Medical equipment can be used to teach, such as mannequins and simulations.
- **Guest speakers**: Physicians, advance practice nurses, social workers, infection control nurses, administrators, risk managers, and substance abuse counselors all may serve as guest speakers.

Educational Needs of Caregivers

The caregiver of the hospice or palliative care patient needs specific education in a number of areas:

- **Stress**: The caregiver should be aware of the indications and effects of stress on the individual, patient, and family members, methods of dealing with stress, and when to ask for help.
- **Community resources**: Needs may be many and varied, and the caregiver often needs assistance from outside agencies.
- **Patient care**: The caregiver should understand basic patient care, such as assisting the patient with bathing, dressing, transferring, and taking/administering medications. The caregiver should also receive education regarding appropriate diet and nutrition, wound care, and any other necessary medical care (such as catheter care).
- **Signs/symptoms of imminent death**: Family members need to know what to expect when death nears, such as increasing incontinence or lack of urinary output and sleeping, death rattle, mottling of skin, Cheyne-Stokes breath, increased confusion, and hallucinations (seeing decreased relatives). This knowledge helps reduce fear and better prepares family members to cope with the changes and to know when to seek help from professional caregivers.
- **End-stage disease progression**: Both the patient and family should be prepared for changes that may occur and should know how to deal with these changes. For example, if a patient is expected to have increased dyspnea, patient and family should be aware of options for oxygen supplementation and optimal positioning to relieve symptoms.
- **Pain and symptom management**: Patients and their families need to understand the patient's right to control of pain and other negative symptoms and should know, step-by-step, how to manage them and what resources are available to help, including medications or other treatments that may alleviate symptoms and any equipment (such as a hospital bed or wheelchair) that may be of use.

Hospice vs. Palliative Care

It is important to be able to educate the patient and family on the differences between hospice care and palliative care.

Hospice care	Palliative care
Duration: Hospice care is intended for the last 6 months of life.	Duration: Palliative care is intended for throughout the illness.
Patients have a terminal medical condition.	Patients have a serious medical condition.
In-home care is covered through Medicare hospice benefit without need for qualifying hospital stay.	In-home treatment is not usually covered by Medicare unless patient has qualifying hospital stay.
Care is usually provided in home environment.	Care is usually provided in inpatient facility but can be provided at home.
Treatment focuses on comfort and pain control and preparation for death.	Treatment focuses on comfort and pain control.
Patients forego life-saving treatment.	Life-saving treatment may continue.
Age: Those qualified for Medicare part A are usually 65 or older, although some insurance plans may provide coverage for younger individuals.	Age: Any age can qualify, although services may or may not be covered by insurance.

Benefit vs. Burden of Treatment Options

Patients and their families must be educated on the benefits and burdens of various treatment options at the end of life.

Treatments	Benefits	Burdens
Hydration	Prevents thirst, prevents drying of mucus membranes, and provides reassurance/comfort to family.	May increase death rattle, increase nausea and vomiting, increase pulmonary and generalized edema, prolong the dying process (minimally) and hasten breakdown of skin.
Turning, repositioning	Prevents pressure sores (although some breakdown of skin may be unavoidable) or worsening of existing sores, helps prevent infection and associated odor and exudate, and prevents contractures.	May increase pain and general discomfort and may be counter to the patient's desire to be left undisturbed, may increase dyspnea when positioned on the side.
Opioid administration	Relieves pain and perception of shortness of breath, and may relieve anxiety and fear of death.	May result in depressed respirations, hallucinations, impaired ability to communicate, loss of consciousness, increased constipation, and a hastening of the dying process.
Resuscitation efforts	Allow family to deny death is imminent.	Cause unnecessary suffering and prolong dying process

Treatments	Benefits	Burdens
Supplemental nutrition	Relieve family's anxiety that the patient is hungry. Prolong life.	May cause nausea, vomiting. May increase tumor growth with cancer. May increase discomfort.
Active treatments (antibiotics, chemotherapy)	Prolong life. Relieve symptoms. Reassure family.	Prolong the dying process. Side effects may be severe (as with chemotherapy).
Glucocorticoids	Reduces intracranial pressure, increases appetite, controls pain, reduces fatigue.	Can result in insomnia, GI upset, delirium, depression, increased risk of infection and hyperglycemia, Cushing's syndrome, anxiety, increased risk of thromboembolism, myopathy, and interference with other medications.

Communication Theory, Principles, and Barriers

Communicating with the Palliative Care Patient and Family

A vital role of the nurse in a palliative care setting is to facilitate **communication** and establish a trusting relationship with the patient and family. Communication takes place on many different levels and the message received may not always be that intended by the sender. In fact, as much as 80% of all communication takes place on the nonverbal level. Though the information can be overwhelming to the patient or family, most individuals expect honesty and truthfulness in their communications with a health care provider. Communication should establish the following: trust and openness, inclusion of the patient and family in all options and care decisions, assurances to the individual and family that they will be listened to and respected, and that they will not be ignored or abandoned. Nurses should avoid and resolve conflicts and allow patients and families to vocalize their needs, expecting them to be addressed. It is also important to extend this communication to the entire health care team to better facilitate understanding and continuity of care.

Communicating about Diagnosis and Progression of Disease

When communicating about a patient's **diagnosis and progression** of disease, the approach and the vocabulary depend on the receiver of the information. When communicating with professionals, such as physicians and other nurses, the information is usually provided in a factual and organized manner, using appropriate medical terminology and common abbreviations. However, when communicating with family members and patients, the nurse must consider the family or patient's age, condition, and ability to understand as well as readiness (physical and emotional) to learn and understand. Communication with the family and patient should always begin with asking what they know and what they want to know, followed by addressing the issues in language that they can understand. It's important to avoid focusing only on medical issues and not considering the emotional impact of information. The nurse should also avoid changing the subject to avoid sensitive discussions.

Adjusting Communication to Receiver Response

Adjusting communication to the receiver's response requires close observation of not only the words of a receiver but also nonverbal responses, such as body language, facial expression, and eye contact. The healthcare provider should avoid giving advice, asking for reasons, patronizing, giving false assurance, interrupting, or trying to force a response. **Common receiver responses** include:

- **Anger**: May be expressed directly or indirectly by criticizing care or particular caregivers or changing physicians. Remain calm, validate concerns, ask what the person needs/wants, and help make a plan for resolution.
- **Shame/guilt**: May be a response to a particular diagnosis, care needs, or belief in culpability. Reassure, express empathy without directly using the word "shame" or "guilt," provide factual information, and avoid all judgmental statements.
- **Fear**: May result from lack of information, bad news, unfamiliarity, or lack of control. Show compassion and empathy, provide clear and appropriate information, reassure, and provide support as needed.
- **Confusion**: May result from emotional overload, medications, and medical condition. Revisit, provide information in simple terms, and reassure.

Advance Care Planning

The nurse must remain attentive to the patient and recognize opportunities to discuss advance care planning, such as when a patient comments or asks questions about the future or prognosis. The discussion should not be hurried, so if necessary the nurse should set a time to have the discussion: "I see you have questions about the future. I'd like to sit down and talk about advance care planning with you this afternoon, if that's all right." A discussion of advance care planning should include:

- What advance planning means
- Cultural attitude toward advance care planning
- Different types of advance care planning
- Legal aspects (including those that are state-specific) and benefits to the patient
- How advance care planning affects treatment
- References for obtaining appropriate advance care documents
- Storing and maintaining advance care documents
- Emotional impact of advance care planning
- Right to opt out of advance care planning or to alter plans

Discussions Related to Resuscitation Efforts

Discussions related to resuscitation efforts are sensitive and should involve not only the patient but also close family members who may be in the position to make decisions if the patient is unable to do so. The patient and the family members may have very different opinions, and this needs to be discussed and resolved. It's important during the discussion about resuscitation to discuss all different aspects, including cardiopulmonary resuscitation, fluid resuscitation, and mechanical ventilation. Patients often believe making decisions about resuscitation is an all-or-nothing proposition; however, patients can specify the types of resuscitation they want. Some patients, for example, may be willing to undergo cardiopulmonary resuscitation efforts but are opposed to being maintained on mechanical ventilation. Any discussion of resuscitation should include the importance of having an advance directive in place although it is not, in fact, legally binding in all states.

Facilitating Patient and Family Conferences

The nurse should be alert to the need for a patient/family conference. Indications include:

- The patient and family have many questions about diagnosis, treatment, or prognosis.
- The patient and family members have differing ideas about end-of-life care.
- The patient will need one or more family members to provide care or other support.
- Family members have unrealistic expectations of the patient or vice versa.
- The patient and family members are involved in conflict.
- The patient and family members fail to communicate effectively.
- The patient or family members appear confused about the patient's condition or care issues.

Depending on the type of concern, the nurse should contact appropriate team members and consultants to participate in the patient/family conference, explaining the rationale for their participation. These members may include a spiritual advisor, physician, physical therapist, nurses, and pharmacist. It's important to elicit as much input as possible from the patient and family members, stressing that the purpose of the conference is to assist rather than direct.

SPIKES Strategy for Providing Sensitive Information

The SPIKES strategy (Beale et al.) can be used as a guide to providing sensitive information (bad news) to the patient and family:

S	**S**et up interview	Make a plan for delivering news and arrange for a private space and presence of significant others (such as spouses or children).
P	Assess patient **p**erception	Question the patient/family about what they know about the disease and discover any misperceptions.
I	Obtain **i**nvitation	Ask the patient/family directly if they want information and how much and respect their decisions, remaining available for questions.
K	Provide **k**nowledge	Provide sensitive information or bad news slowly rather than quickly so the patient and family have time to digest the information. Ask if they have questions and avoid technical jargon. Consider psychosocial implications as well as cultural differences.
E	Address **e**motions	Respond to the patient's/family's feelings and emotional response. Attempt to identify emotional response (sad, depressed, angry, confused) and acknowledge (move closer, touch patient, express regret, verbally respond).
S	**S**trategy/ **S**ummary	Ask if the patient and family are ready to discuss a treatment plan. Present treatment options if "yes" and set up a later time to discuss if "no."

Use of Interpreters

Healthcare agencies that are federally funded are required to provide free **interpretive services** for clients speaking commonly encountered foreign languages. The patient must be informed that an interpreter will be made available to them. In order to ensure appropriate care and communication, a third-party interpreter who is trained in medical terminology, fluent in both languages being used, and is familiar with the ethics and HIPAA regulations of acting as an interpreter is the best option. Meeting these requirements ensures compliance with federal guidelines. Family members cannot be required to serve as interpreters unless the client specifically requests a family member to act in this capacity. In emergency situations it is appropriate to use whatever means are readily available to assist in communicating with the patient.

Family and Caregiver Support

Caregiver Support in Terminal Illness

The nurse must understand that terminal illness and death involve the entire family. The family's response to an illness will depend on the stage of life that they are in as well as the basic family relationships and dynamics. Nurses should help reduce both physical and emotional burdens placed on the **caregiver** and other family members. They should provide the knowledge and skills needed to enhance the patient's comfort. The nurse should also provide access to additional caregiver support resources. Interventions and referrals might include respite care, social worker assistance, occupational therapy, and referrals to help simplify tasks and conserve energy, along with referral for an aide to help with patient ADLs. The nurse is responsible for frequent assessment of the caregiver's health and his or her ability to provide care, as well as watching for signs of neglect and abuse. The nurse strives to help the family develop healthy ways to cope as they prepare for the impending death.

Caregiver Assessment and Interventions

Assessing caregiver ability begins with asking the caregiver about the skills the person has, what the caregiver feels comfortable doing, and what areas the caregiver needs assistance. This shows respect for the caregiver and allows the caregiver to express concerns. The best method of assessing the actual **skills** is to work with the caregiver and observe, providing positive feedback during the process. Rather than criticizing ("Don't pull your spouse under the arms"), a better approach is focus on the caregiver's needs ("Let me show you how to move your spouse without risking injuring your back"). Assessment should include not only the caregiver's knowledge and physical ability to provide care but also the caregiver's **emotional ability, resources available, values, and perceptions**. It's important to know if the caregiver is willing to provide care or is doing so out of necessity, as this may affect the caregiver's sense of wellbeing and the patient-caregiver relationship.

Promoting Family Self-Care Activities

The nurse can promote family self-care activities by:

- Assessing the need for care and the strengths and weaknesses of the family
- Educating the family about the burdens and benefits of provision of care
- Providing demonstrations and practice to help the family gain confidence in provision of care
- Engaging the patient and family in development of the plan of care so they feel some degree of control
- Serving as a mentor and resource for the family
- Modeling appropriate care
- Educating the family about the importance of personal time and respite
- Providing information about respite services
- Assisting family with coping strategies, such as relaxation and visualization
- Discussing risks for increased stress, such as inadequate sleep, poor diet, lack of exercise, and failure to care for personal health issues
- Assisting family members to set personal goals (such as taking a daily walk or nap)
- Helping family create a problem list and possible solutions

Caregiver Fatigue

Caregiver fatigue is very common and can relate to physical or emotional fatigue. The nurse should discuss issues of **caregiver fatigue** early in the care process if possible so that the caregiver is aware of the effects of stress and overwork. Caregivers often get inadequate sleep and become exhausted from the constant demands of patient care and have no idea where to turn for help. The nurse should address signs of fatigue directly ("You look exhausted") to encourage the caregiver to discuss problems. If the patient is under hospice care and is eligible for respite care, the nurse can help to facilitate this. The nurse can also provide the caregiver with information about community resources that may help to reduce the burden of care, such as Meals-on-Wheels, volunteers, adult day care, and caregiver support groups, and should assess the environment to determine if accommodations would be helpful.

Caregiver Support Programs

Home Meal Delivery Programs

Home meal delivery programs (such as Meals-on-Wheels) provide nutritious meals for homebound adults (often restricted to older adults). The programs usually serve meals 5-7 days a week with home delivery, often by volunteers. Meals are usually low cost ($2-4 per meal) but this varies with program. Most programs deliver one hot meal a day and may provide food for one or two other meals (such as a sandwich for dinner and cold cereal for breakfast the next day). Requirements and age restrictions vary with some serving those ≥60 and others ≥65. People with temporary disabilities may be restricted in length of service. Some programs are intended for those with low incomes, but others do not have income restrictions. Most programs provide little choice in menu but may offer low fat, low salt, or low carbohydrate diets. Many home meal delivery programs have waiting lists because the need outpaces the number of programs.

Home Health Agencies

Home health agencies provide intermittent care in the home environment or assisted-living facilities. Home health care can include nursing care (assessment, medications, and treatment), social workers, speech pathologists, physical and occupational therapists, and certified nurse aides (personal care). Home health agencies may provide professionals to draw blood for lab tests and administer intravenous fluids. Home health care allows patients to be sent home earlier from acute hospitals and skilled nursing facilities and is more cost effective than in-patient care. Many Home Health Agencies include hospice care. Some insurance companies pay for home health care, and Medicare pays for care with requirements: Patients must be homebound, in need of skilled care <7 days/week or <8 hours each day over a period of ≤21 days. Those eligible may receive home health aide services, but total hours of care may not exceed 28-35 hours/week (depending on need). Medicare pays a set amount for each episode of care (60-day period), depending on the health care condition.

Adult Daycare

Adult daycare is an option to provide caregiver respite and to allow caregivers to continue with employment. Daycare programs are generally intended for older adults who require some type of supervision and/or assistance. The focus of daycare programs may be on:

- Social interaction
- Medical assistance
- Alzheimer care

Most adult daycare programs have some type of nursing supervision and nursing care to assist with toileting, medications, eating, walking, and social activities and are open during usual daytime hours (such as from 8 AM to 5 PM) and provide 1 or 2 meals and snacks, sometimes at extra cost. Costs may vary widely, with costs typically higher for those that provide specialized services. Costs are usually not covered by health insurance or Medicare although some long-term care policies may provide coverage. If the program is licensed as an Alzheimer's program, Medicaid may cover some costs.

Psychosocial Issues at the End of Life

MALADAPTIVE BEHAVIORS

Six maladaptive behaviors that patients and families dealing with life-threatening illnesses may exhibit are:

- **Denial**: A way for the person to reject the reality of the situation they find themselves in. It is a refusal to accept physical, psychological, and emotional knowledge they do not want to believe in or deal with. Denial may be transiently adaptive when it is brief, securing only a little more time to gather the emotional reserves necessary for successful coping.
- **Guilt**: An unreasonable feeling of responsibility for negative influences or consequences over which the person may or may not have control.
- **Depression**: A mental state of hopelessness and despair. A severe loss of happiness and motivation.
- **Avoidance**: Withdrawal or turning away from actions or consequences associated with negative stimuli.
- **Decathexis**: Withdrawing prior feelings of affection for and attachment to a person or object, typically in anticipation of an impending loss.
- **Aggression**: Hostile behavior, whether physical or verbal, meant to be demeaning, destructive and increase negative emotions in those around them.

MANAGING EMOTIONAL STATES IN PATIENTS

DENIAL AND ANGER/HOSTILITY

Denial and anger/hostility are very common first reactions to bad news, and some patients are unable to get past these emotional states:

- **Denial**: Patients may act stunned and immobile or detached and unable to respond appropriately. In the beginning, denial serves as a protective mechanism that allows the patient to cope, but as time passes patients may become increasingly resistive to information and treatment, attempting to carry on as though everything is normal or blaming symptoms on minor problems, such as "heart burn." The nurse should remain patient and supportive, and repeat information as many times as needed while avoiding forcing the patient to "face the truth."
- **Anger and/or hostility**: Some patients may lash out at others and express overt hostility. Others may blame themselves or others for their conditions. Some patients are resentful they are ill and may complain loudly and often about medical care and healthcare providers. The nurse must not respond in anger or take patient statements personally but should remain calm and supportive while alert to the risk of physical attack.

FEAR

Fear is a common feeling among hospice and palliative care patients, and while some fears may be irrational, many are realistic, so identifying the patient's fear and developing strategies to alleviate those fears are important to the patient's sense of wellbeing:

Fears	Strategies
Pain	Maintaining adequate pain control and preventing breakthrough pain is essential, as is giving the patient some degree of control over decisions about pain control.
Treatments	Provide accurate information about what treatments entail and what type of discomfort and adverse effects to expect, especially in relation to surgery, chemotherapy, and radiotherapy.
Change of self-image	Provide patients with information about expected physical changes (loss of hair, amputation, scars) and prostheses (wigs, breast prosthesis, limb prosthesis) and other methods (clothing, makeup) to disguise or modify physical changes.
Costs	Provide information about costs and resources for financial and other assistance.
Dependency	Encourage the patient to remain independent in decisions or care to the degree possible and provide emotional support to the patient and caregiver.
Dying	Encourage the patient to express feelings and carry out a life review.

GUILT

Guilt is a common emotion associated with hospice and/or palliative care:

- **Patients** often feel guilty about leaving family behind. They may regret actions that they have taken or failed to take and feel guilty about being a burden, especially if they depend on family for caregiving, and about the cost of care. The nurse should take time to listen to the patient and help the patient focus on positive things the patient has provided for the family.
- **Family members** may feel that they have not done enough to help or may begin to regret harsh thoughts or things they have said. They may wish the patient would die to end suffering or relieve them from caregiving, but then feel guilty about wishing the patient's death. Some may feel guilty about placing a patient in hospice care or that they were not present when the patient died. The nurse should listen and support the family, reassuring them that the feelings that they have experienced are normal and that it's not unusual for patients to wait until family are gone to die. Some may benefit from a support group.

ANXIETY

Peplau's four levels of anxiety include:

1. **Mild**: Feelings include increased motivation, sharpened senses, alertness, enlarged perceptual field, restlessness, irritability, and hypersensitivity to sensory input, but the client can still solve problems, and learning is effective. Client may experience GI upset ("butterflies").
2. **Moderate**: The perceptual field narrows to a specific task and attention is selective. The client speaks rapidly in a high pitch and experiences muscle tension, diaphoresis, pounding pulse, headache, dry mouth, GI upset, and frequent urination.

3. **Severe**: The perceptual field continues to narrow, and the client cannot complete tasks, solve problems, or learn effectively. The client feels fear, dread, or horror and experiences severe headache, GI upset, trembling, rigidity, vertigo, pallor, tachycardia, and chest pain. Actions may be ritualistic.
4. **Panic**: Perceptual field focuses on self, not responding to environmental stimuli. The client experiences perceptual distortions, is unable to think rationally or recognize danger, and may be suicidal. The client may have disorganized personality, delusions, hallucinations, and inability to speak. The client may run or remain immobile.

SUFFERING

There are multiple aspects of **suffering** in which an individual can feel pain or distress. It encompasses emotional, spiritual, and physical aspects of life and affects the whole person. Suffering must be addressed from a comprehensive, holistic perspective while recognizing that it is not always possible to find the source, or entirely resolve all suffering. Identifying suffering involves careful observation, and different disciplinary perspectives can be helpful in making an accurate assessment. Issues surrounding suffering must be adequately addressed or the suffering is more likely to compound rather than diminish over time. However, it is not necessary for the caregiver to give, or even have, answers to the difficult questions that may arise. Rather, the primary intervention requires in reassurance of non-abandonment and continued support while the patient seeks answers for themselves. Religious or spiritual counseling is often useful as well.

HOPE

Multiple factors can affect an individual's **outlook during a terminal illness**. Among these are the opportunity and ability to experience one or more meaningful relationships. All individuals need to feel that they are needed and an important part of the lives of their loved ones. Maintaining contact with family and close friends is thus crucial. In addition, maintaining feelings of lightheartedness, delight, joy, or playfulness will also help the individual identify and express positive personal attributes. They will be more accepting of themselves and others if they are able to identify courage, determination, serenity, and positive esteem within themselves. Spiritual beliefs and participation in spiritual rituals can provide a further sense of meaning to their life. The individual can thereby better focus their energies on achieving short-term, positive goals by which to provide direction to their lives, and allowing them to continue to share meaningfully with others. In the final stages of a terminal illness, individuals who have maintained a feeling of hope and other positive feelings are able to look toward their eventual death with greater peace and serenity.

In assessing whether or not an individual is experiencing exaggerated or unrealistic hope, determine if the hope is either too broad or too dismissive in nature, such as a complete denial of the disease process itself or a persistent belief in a cure when none is available. If the hope is unlikely to be realized, how determined is the individual to their course of belief? Is he or she able to acknowledge the possibility of a negative outcome? Or does the individual claim a sure knowledge of what will happen, rather than expressing realistic hopes and fears? Those experiencing unrealistic hope are more likely to engage in reckless behaviors and to ignore or dismiss worsening symptoms or warning signs. Such unrealistic hope may alienate the individual from family and friends, ultimately creating isolation. Is the person's level of hope impeding their ability to place their personal affairs in order or to acknowledge and properly grieve their own loss? Realistic hope allows for the wish of a miracle, even while preparing for the likelihood of a loss. Realistic hope becomes more, rather than less, accepting over time.

Coping Mechanisms

Coping mechanisms are important for people to deal effectively with stress (often associated with loss), and those who have overcome trauma and/or loss over the course of their lifetime tend to utilize the most effective strategies. Those with ineffective coping skills may express anxiety, anger, and agitation (which may interfere with decision making) and may develop depression and physical ailments, such as anorexia, weight loss, nausea, urinary and bowel problems, and sleep disturbance. **Coping mechanisms** include:

- **Avoidance**: Finding means to avoid stressors or reduce their impact is sometimes possible.
- **Problem solving**: Actively searching for a way to reduce stress or cope with it can promote self-assurance.
- **Physical activity**: An exercise program can often increase feelings of wellbeing and allow people to cope more effectively.
- **Spirituality**: About 90% of older adults are religious, with 50% attending religious services, and religion/spiritual endeavors can provide emotional support and a positive outlook to help people cope.

Task-Oriented Coping

Some people cope best with dying by focusing on the tasks that must be completed throughout the process. These **tasks** may be summarized as follows:

- **Physical tasks**: Bodily needs must be met and physical distress minimized in ways that are consistent with the patient's values and beliefs.
- **Psychological tasks**: The patient must feel a sense of dignity. They will seek reassurance and satisfaction in their lives, as well as security and autonomy.
- **Social tasks**: Interpersonal relationships must be nurtured and sustained, and past conflicts resolved and forgiveness expressed in order to fully address the social and relational implications of dying.
- **Spiritual tasks**: Sources of spiritual energy must be identified, developed, and reaffirmed in order to secure a continuing hope and purpose to their existence.

COPING ASSISTANCE

Many factors influence a patient's coping abilities, including the patient's disability, socio-demographic characteristics, personality, and the social and physical environment. Patients who lack self-efficacy (belief in one's abilities to cope) and hope may have difficulty coping or may utilize coping strategies, such as avoidance, that may be counterproductive. **Coping assistance** may include:

- Educating the patient about coping strategies
- Helping the patient come to terms with the condition through encouraging patient to share experiences and through active listening
- Utilizing strategies to promote self-awareness (education, feedback, counseling, rating tasks)
- Providing positive reinforcement
- Providing opportunities for the patient to make decisions and to be as independent as possible
- Helping the patient to establish order in his or her life through pacing, planning, and prioritizing
- Providing a home-based education program for the patient and family
- Encouraging small successes to help instill hope
- Enhancing support systems through encouraging friends and family to participate in rehabilitation
- Establishing a therapeutic relationship with the patient

SUICIDAL IDEATION

Patients with chronic and/or terminal illnesses are at increased risk of **suicidal ideation** because they no longer want to live with pain, they do not want to become or remain a burden to family, they do not want to become dependent on others, they are lonely and frightened, they are exhausted from caregiving, and/or they suffer from depression or mood disorders.

- **Passive suicidal ideation** involves wishing to be dead or thinking about dying without making plans while active suicidal ideation involves making plans.
- Those with **active suicidal ideation** are most at risk. People with suicidal ideation often give signals, direct or indirect, to indicate they are considering suicide because many people have some ambivalence and want help. They may, for example, have a sudden change in mood, talk about dying, begin to give things away, stop taking medications, and/or become increasingly withdrawn. Others may act impulsively or effectively hide their distress.

A **suicide risk assessment** should be completed and documented upon admission, with each shift change, at discharge, or any time suicidal ideation is suggested by the individual. Interventions include asking the patient about suicidal ideation, discussing feelings, making a safety plan, treating pain more effectively, and helping to resolve problems.

Sleep Disturbances

Sleep disturbances are common among hospice and palliative care patients, especially those with cancer, and may be associated with anxiety and depression, medications (corticosteroids, chemotherapeutic agents), pain, and other medical conditions (ALS, obstructive or central sleep apnea, restless legs syndrome, diabetes, arthritis, CHF, coronary artery disease, GERD, asthma, thyroid disorders, and renal failure). **Insomnia** is most common although some patients (especially those depressed) may sleep excessively and remain **somnolent**. Management begins by identifying and treating the underlying cause when possible:

- **Pharmacologic treatment**: Includes benzodiazepines (estazolam, quazepam, temazepam, flurazepam, lorazepam, triazolam), non-benzodiazepine receptor agonists (zaleplon, zolpidem, eszopiclone), melatonin-receptor agonist (ramelteon), and tricyclic antidepressants (amitriptyline, doxepin, mirtazapine, trazadone).
- **Non-pharmacologic treatment**: Includes exercise regimens, cognitive-behavioral therapy, education about the effects of medication, and complementary therapies, such as aromatherapy, massage, self-hypnosis, mindfulness, and relaxation and visualization exercises. Some patients may benefit from better sleep hygiene and resetting the sleep-wake cycle by avoiding excessive napping or taking a short daily nap, setting a regular time for sleep, limiting fluid intake before bed (if nocturia present), avoiding caffeine in the afternoon and evening, and keeping the bedroom quiet and peaceful.

Intimacy/Relationship Issues

Intimacy/relationship issues may arise between hospice and palliative care patients and their significant others:

- **Dynamics of dependency**: Role reversal may occur as the person who was previously dominant (such as the primary wage earner) may become dependent on the other person for financial support and/or caregiving. This may cause guilt, resentment, depression, and anger (on both parts). A stay-at-home parent may have to seek employment, and this can become stressful, especially if the person lacks marketable skills.
- **Impotence, decreased libido**: Pain, medications, progression of disease, and depression can all impair the patient's interest in or ability to engage in sexual intercourse.
- **Lack of privacy**: Patients who are hospitalized in an acute, long-term care, or hospice facility often have little privacy, especially if they share a room with another patient.

The nurse should discuss intimacy/relationship issues with patients and significant others, encouraging them to express their feelings and providing resources, including information about alternative methods of expressing intimacy, such as through cuddling, massage, or oral sex. When possible, the nurse should assist the patient to achieve some privacy, such as through bed curtains or signs on the door.

Cultural Issues

Each person is entitled to receive an individualized full assessment and personalized care. The nurse should first assess his or her own background, values, and beliefs in order to consciously avoid placing biases upon the patient. Obtain further knowledge in order to understand the background of the patient being addressed, and show acceptance of differences even when they may diverge from the nurse's own comfort zone and culture. Nurses should also acknowledge differences concerning end-of life care and be sensitive and open to the individual patient's beliefs rather than trying to predict behavior or impose ideas. Assumptions regarding care, needs, or beliefs should not be made based on assumptions arising from a patient's race or ethnicity.

Culture is a set of learned and shared experiences among a group and is continuously changing. Culture is not based on heredity or genes. Culture may guide behavior, but not all members of a group follow the same cultural traditions or beliefs. Members of a cultural group may have divergent personal beliefs that are variations of the whole tradition. Individuals become members of a cultural group when they adopt the group's basic beliefs and values. Smaller groups may realign themselves with a larger or more dominate culture through **acculturation**. **Ethnicity** describes a similarity in ancestry, history, and/or language that a group has in common. Members of an ethnic group may share social, political, and cultural backgrounds. Not everyone who shares ethnicity will relate to or feel they belong with the rest of the group. Ethnic groups can house several different cultural groups. **Race** is a term often used to define human differences through genetic and biological means, but it is not scientifically supported.

Culturally competent behavior goes beyond knowing general culture-based facts; it is a dynamic process of being aware of and showing respect for cultural differences of all types. It begins with being aware of one's own beliefs and not letting them interfere with the care provided. Just as each nurse brings his or her own individual background, beliefs and practices to the caring experience, each patient and family has their own unique contributions to the world and environment of the care plan. Cultural competence is providing knowledgeable care that corresponds with the patient and family's own cultural background. The nurse provides a complete and unbiased, sensitive assessment of the patient's background and beliefs, obtains further knowledge as necessary, then coordinates and executes a plan of care that is meaningful to the patient and the family regardless of the care provider's own beliefs.

C. M. Fong proposed the mnemonic **CONFHER** to summarize an assessment model to ensure culturally sensitive care.

- Communication: Identify the patient's primary language and comprehension level.
- Orientation: Ask to whom the patient relates. Find out their ethnic identity and identify their value orientations and acculturation.
- Nutrition: Find out the patient's food preferences and restrictions. Ask the patient about their feelings, associations, and meanings behind food.
- Family relationships: Identify the family structure, dynamics, and goals.
- Health and health beliefs: Discuss the patient's personal beliefs and health behaviors.
- Education: Identify the patient's cognitive style. Find out about their formal education, occupation, or profession.
- Religion: Discuss the patient's spiritual beliefs and practices. Find out if the patient relates to a higher power and if they have a religious preference.

Grief, Loss, and Bereavement

Basic Tenets in Relation to Death and Dying

Roman Catholicism

Roman Catholics often pray with a rosary and may ask for the Sacrament of the Sick. Symbols such as crosses, holy water, and pictures and statues of saints hold significance.

Orthodox/Conservative Judaism

After death, the body is cleaned and wrapped in a linen shroud. Embalming is considered a desecration of the body, and cremation is never done because the body must contact the earth, and the body is never displayed. Family should be with the patient at the time of death and the body should be attended while awaiting burial, and those in attendance should not eat or drink in the presence of the body. Mourning practices are carried out to comfort the living and demonstrate respect for the dead. Organ donation is permitted and considered a good deed.

Judaism

For a Jewish patient, all mirrors should be covered at the time of death. A prayer for the dead, called the Kaddish, is recited and the body receives a special washing. There is an urgency to complete the burial process within 24 hours of the death. This should occur before sundown in that same time frame. The only exception is if it interferes with Sabbath. The Jewish faith also observes *shiva*— the seven-day grieving period after the burial of a loved one. During this time the mourners do not work. Mourning for a parent lasts one year. Kosher foods are required.

Hinduism

After death, the body is cleansed and adorned. Cremation is practiced to free the soul from the body and the existence on earth. However, unnamed babies and untouchables (low caste) have traditionally been buried. Individuals may decide about organ donation. Hindus believe the soul experiences many lifetimes and that life unfolds according to *karma.*

Buddhism

Buddhists believe that the soul stays with the body for some time after death, so family members may wish to leave the deceased undisturbed for a period of time to allow the soul time to leave the body in peace. Buddhists believe that the soul experiences multiple lifetimes to learn necessary lessons and that actions in a previous lifetime influence the current life, including illnesses, and that death is a natural part of the transition from one life to another. Buddhists are usually cremated. Individuals may decide about organ donation.

Islam

Islamic tradition forbids cremation of the body or embalming. Traditionally, the body is bathed with water (with genitals covered) usually by members of the family who are of the same gender or are a spouse or parent of a minor child. The body is then wrapped in a shroud, usually plain white cloth with 3 pieces used for males and 5 for females. Funeral prayers (*Janazah*) are said during a gathering of people to honor the dead. Burial should be within 24 hours and to at least a depth of 5 feet. Organ donation is generally permitted.

RANDO'S SIX R'S

Rando (1984) described **six active grieving tasks** ("grief work") of the bereaved. The six Rs include:

- **Recognizing**: The person must recognize the degree of loss and accept that the loss is real.
- **Reacting**: The person actively experiences the emotional response to the loss.
- **Recollecting and re-experiencing**: The person reviews memories of the person who has died, re-experiencing events.
- **Relinquishing**: The person accepts that the loss has caused the world to change and that there is no return from that reality.
- **Readjusting**: The person begins to grieve less, returning to daily life and feeling less overwhelmed with loss.
- **Reinvesting**: The person accepts the changes that the loss has brought and begins to actively reenter the world, form new associations and relationships, and make new commitments.

BEREAVEMENT

Bereavement occurs after the death of a family member, friend, or someone to whom a person identifies closely. It is a time of mourning and is part of the natural grieving process, but some people are not able to move past the grieving process and may suffer signs related to severe depression, such as poor appetite, insomnia, and other symptoms, such as chest pain, that may mimic physical illnesses. Some may enter a stage of denial or anger that interferes with their daily activities and work. People suffering bereavement may present with vague and varied complaints. A careful history is important. Treatment varies according to the needs of the individual. In some cases, SSRIs (such as Prozac) may provide temporary relief, but the client should be referred for psychological counseling, bereavement services, or psychiatric care, depending upon the severity of symptoms.

ASSESSING FOR COMPLICATED BEREAVEMENT

Families should be assessed for the risk of **complicated bereavement**, which may indicate the need for counseling to help individuals cope. Complicated bereavement can result in prolonged periods of mourning, depression, and negative impacts of social interactions and health. Risk assessment begins with family interview and may include specific tools, such as the Bereavement Experience Questionnaire, and the Bereavement Risk Index. Indications that a person is undergoing traumatic grief include a duration of at least 60 days of the following:

- Avoiding reminders of or talking about the deceased
- Exhibiting signs of depression and negative feelings about the future
- Feeling numb, dazed, shocked
- Having feelings of incompleteness, as though part of self has also died
- Expressing anger, bitterness, and blame associated with the death
- Withdrawing from social or occupational roles
- Exhibiting impaired functioning (careless dress, cluttered home, poor hygiene)
- Losing sense of trust in others and security
- Assuming negative behaviors (smoking, drinking) of the deceased

Factors that Influence Bereavement Process

Factors that influence the bereavement process include:

- **Type of death**: Sudden unexpected death can be much harder to cope with than death after an extended chronic illness during which the bereaved has had time to come to terms with the fact that the patient is dying. Suicide can be especially traumatic because the bereaved may have feelings of guilt or may anguish over failing to save the person.
- **Support system**: Bereaved who lacks a strong support system may be unable to express feelings or come to terms with them.
- **Age of bereaved**: Young people may feel abandoned and angry while older people may focus on feelings of loneliness and loss.
- **Secondary losses**: Death may mean a sudden loss of income (such as with the death of the head of a household) or a sudden increase in responsibilities (need to get a job, necessity of maintaining a home and caring for children alone). Friendships may falter.

Life Completion and Closure

Developmental landmarks associated with **life completion and closure** include:

- A sense of completion in all affairs, including worldly, community, and interpersonal relationships with family and friends. The individual must feel that they have taken care of all unfinished business.
- They feel a satisfaction in life and work. After reflecting on their lives, patients can accept themselves and their accomplishments as fulfilling and worthwhile.
- They can experience feelings of love and acceptance for self and others: pursuing worthiness, forgiveness, gratitude, closure, and resolution of past hurts and wrongs to bring about peace and satisfaction.
- The patient is able to identify a general understanding of the meaning and finality of life.
- They express a willingness to move forward into the unknown, accepting death and saying goodbye.

Visual Life Review Projects

When the patient is ready for a life review, the nurse can suggest that he or she begins by looking at **old photos** and **home movies**. These are often a source of happiness and encourage recitation of memories and favorite times during family life. Most people are apt to take photographs of happy times. Provide a photo album or scrapbook for the patient and family to put together. The album offers an opportunity for patients to relive fond memories with the family, and they can review it independently when family and friends are unavailable. Life review is also helpful for the family after the patient has died. Remember that very young children think death is reversible, and may need to be reminded again and again that someone in the pictures is not coming back. Emphasize that the person who died did not go away because they were angry with the child, and that the doctors could not prevent the death.

Journaling or Telling a Life Story

The end-stage patient and family need to review their life together to identify its meaning. Obtain a **journal** and writing materials for the patient. If the patient wants newspaper clippings to include in the journal, contact a librarian about how to obtain them. The patient may initially be hesitant to review his or her life with others, but as trust is built, will probably do so willingly. Ask the family for their assistance because they shared many of the events with the patient and may have supplemental information. Use the hospice's program resources and guides to assist the patient and family in capturing their memories. If the patient is too weak to write, borrow a tape recorder or get a volunteer to take dictation. The patient may want to preserve favorite memories as a gift for family members, or write explanations, and this is therapeutic for all concerned.

Legacy Interventions at End-of-Life

Legacy interventions are those that promote a life review on the part of the patient at the end-of-life and create a memory product for survivors. **Legacy interventions** include:

- **Encouraging life talk**: The patient and family talk about the patient's life, such as favorite activities, vacations, friends, and special memories.
- Providing **artistic opportunities**: The patient and family can share feelings/memories through drawings, paintings, and music.
- Creating a **scrapbook**: This may include pictures, drawings, certificates, diplomas, awards, and other things that are important to the patient.
- Creating a **video journal or audiotape journal**: A smart phone or other video/audio recording device may be used to record messages to family members or memories.
- **Story/poetry writing**: Some patients may want to write a story or poem that expresses their feelings.
- Making **handprints or fingerprint jewelry**: Kits are available to save handprints of children, and a fingerprint can be memorialized in silver or other metal.

Creating an Audio or Video Legacy

End-stage patients want to ascribe meaning to their lives. Life review happens in most cultures. Ask a librarian to inspire the patient with an autobiography from an author with the same cultural and spiritual background. If the patient wishes to leave an **audio legacy**, obtain the resources from the recreation director or occupational therapist. Schedule recording for a time when the patient has the most energy and will be able to participate fully. If the patient desires to create a video for family or friends, make certain the patient is groomed appropriately. Find out how to disguise illness with makeup through Look Good Feel Better, which donates complimentary tool kits and teaches patients how to use hair alternatives, prosthetic clothing, and cosmetics. Help the patient call family members or friends to arrange a film debut. If they cannot attend in person, ask the IT manager how to broadcast the movie over an internet connection.

Phone Calls and Internet Chats

End-stage patients may miss family and friends who do not live locally, or are unable to be physically present. Facilitate communication between the patient and family members or friends because saying a final goodbye is psychologically important for closure. Modern technology makes long-distance communication simple, while requiring little energy expenditure from the patient, and the instantaneous communication brings much comfort. If the patient does not have their own communication devices, arrange time for the patient to use one of facility's devices to communicate with family and friends, ideally corresponding to the time of day when the patient has the most energy, even if that means interrupting the patient's usual schedule.

Patient's and Family's Search for Meaning and Hope

Cultures and families vary in how they perceive illness and disability, and this may profoundly affect the patient's **search for meaning and hope**. It's important to understand the patient's cultural belief system about what causes disease or disability. Likewise, it's important to know how to respond and to show respect for traditions, such as the use of healers. Some cultures attach stigma to some types of diseases, and these attitudes may be difficult to overcome if they are not acknowledged. The patient's family, spiritual, and cultural values should be incorporated into the plan of care. Family members may experience severe stress resulting from the patient's impairment and should be included whenever possible in care decisions and interventions and allowed to express their own feelings of loss and concern. All family members are impacted when one member faces impairment, and family systems may be strained if members are not adequately prepared for helping or caring for the patient, especially after discharge.

Strategies that help the patient/family manage disease and find meaning and hope include:

- **Coaching**: Nurses acting as coaches are responsible for assisting patients to obtain the information and confidence they need to participate actively in the management of their own healthcare. The coach works in collaboration with the patient to provide support in self-management as well as emotional support. The coach conducts follow-ups with the patient and helps the patient navigate the healthcare system.
- **Motivating**: The nurse can encourage patients to change behavior by appealing to their own sense of motivation. Motivating may include the use of motivational interviewing, which focuses on establishing an empathetic relationship with the patient and utilizes open-ended (yes/no) questions, affirmations (expression of empathy), reflective listening, and summary.
- **Negotiating**: It is important to take the time to deliberate with a patient to determine the best course of action. The nurse should present the pros and cons of treatment and provide clear explanations as to why a particular treatment may be indicated, taking into consideration the needs, desires, and concerns of the patient.

Professionalism

Principles of Biomedical Ethics

Promoting Autonomy

Autonomy is the ethical principle that the individual has the right to make decisions about his or her own care. In the case of children or patients with dementia who cannot make autonomous decisions, parents or family members may serve as the legal decision maker. The right of patients to make decisions about end-of-life care through advance directives, to refuse care, and to make informed consent was formalized in the Patient's Self-Determination Act (1991). However, with hospice and palliative care, the nurse must encourage active participation by patients and families and respect cultural differences that may impact decision-making. In some cultures, decisions are often made by the family or the head of the family rather than the individual. Additionally, there are limitations to autonomy. In most states, even if patients want physician-assisted suicide, the practice is illegal.

Decision-Making Models

Do no harm	This model is based on nonmaleficence, the requirement that the treatment provided does no harm; however, by their nature, some treatments can and often do harm patients, so the underlying intent and goal of treatment must be considered when making decisions. For example, CPR may be carried out to save a patient's life and done with correct technique but still result in rib fractures.
In good faith	The motive for a decision should be honest and fair and decisions made with sincere intention to do good even though the outcome may be negative. For example, EMS personnel may provide a treatment for a patient in good faith although the treatment later proves to be ineffective.
Patient's best interest	Making a decision in the patient's best interests includes considering the patient's or parents' (in the case of children) wishes, the best clinical judgment, the best choice of various options, the chances for improvement or decline, and religious or cultural preferences.

Promoting Beneficence

Beneficence is an ethical principle that involves performing actions that are for the purpose of benefitting another person. In the care of a patient, any procedure or treatment should be done with the ultimate goal of benefitting the patient, and any actions that are not beneficial should be reconsidered. While hospice and palliative care focuses on comfort needs rather than extension of life, all of the patient's needs must be considered. Beneficence applies not only to obligatory acts (such as medical treatments) but also to non-obligatory acts (such as taking time to sit and talk with a patient). The patients' physical needs and emotional needs should have equal importance in the provision of care. The nurse has a responsibility to promote beneficence in all aspects of the care plan and to actively work to prevent harm.

Promoting Veracity

Veracity refers to the obligation the healthcare provider has to tell patients and families the truth and to avoid lying or making misleading statements. The nurse should not purposefully withhold information that the patient is entitled to, such as when a medication or treatment error has occurred, although the reality is that patients are often not informed about such occurrences. In Western culture, the idea that people are entitled to truthful information about their condition is paramount and supported by law, but not all cultures view veracity in the same manner. In some cultures, bad news, such as a diagnosis of cancer, is routinely withheld from patients and telling them is considered cruel. The nurse should consider the cultural implications of veracity and discuss the issue with the patient and family members when appropriate, keeping in mind that although truth may be negative it should never be unkind.

Promoting Nonmaleficence

Nonmaleficence is an ethical principle that means healthcare workers should provide care in a manner that does not cause direct intentional harm to the patient:

- The actual act must be good or morally neutral.
- The intent must be only for a good effect.
- A bad effect cannot serve as the means to get to a good effect.
- A good effect must have more benefit than a bad effect has harm.

With provision of care to hospice and palliative care patients, the nurse must continually reevaluate patient care and treatments that may be beneficial initially but later negatively impact the patient's comfort needs. Nonmaleficence is a consideration when patients are receiving chemotherapy or radiotherapy that results in severe adverse effects. These effects must be balanced against the potential for long-term improvement in condition or prolonged survival, considering the patient's wishes.

Promoting Justice

Justice is the ethical principle that relates to the distribution of the limited resources of healthcare benefits to the members of society. This issue may arise when there are more patients than can be accommodated. Decisions should be made according to what is best or most just for the patients and not colored by personal bias. The nurse should apply the principle of justice in ensuring that all patients have equal consideration of their needs and that resources are distributed fairly; however, the realities of healthcare access (insured versus uninsured) present a challenge to upholding justice as some people can afford necessary care and others cannot. The nurse has a responsibility to try to compensate by helping people finding additional sources of financial assistance and supplies that they cannot otherwise afford. Some hospice and palliative care programs have fund raising programs so they can serve patients who lack adequate insurance and/or income.

Policies Regarding Donation of Organs and Tissue

People of any age can donate organs and/or tissue, including organs, stem cells, blood/platelets, tissue, and whole body. There are different types of **donations**:

- **Whole body**: Usually organs cannot be donated separately and the body is donated intact.
- **Donation after cardiac or brain death**: Solid organs must be transplanted 6-72 hours after removal although tissues can be frozen and banked.

Tissues and organs are screened for diseases that may infect the recipient. People who are HIV positive are restricted from donating. Some restrictions apply to patients who die of cancer although some organs can be donated if the cancer hasn't spread within the previous year. Patients with metastasis, primary cerebral lymphoma, or hematologic cancers cannot donate. People may indicate they wish to be organ donors, but family members often must make the decision after patient death. The request for donor organs should be made with sensitivity, and no one should be coerced into approving donation.

Suicidal Ideation

Suicidal ideation occurs frequently in patients with mood disorders or depression. While females are more likely to attempt suicide, males actually commit 3 times more suicides than female, primarily because females tend to take overdoses from which they can be revived while males choose more violent means, such as jumping from a high place, shooting, or hanging. Risk factors include psychiatric disorders (schizophrenia, bipolar disorder, PTSD, substance abuse, and BPD), physical disorders (HIV/AIDS, cancer, diabetes, stroke, traumatic brain injury, and spinal cord injury). Passive suicidal ideation involves wishing to be dead or thinking about dying without making plans while active suicidal ideation involves making plans. Those with active suicidal ideation are most at risk. People with suicidal ideation often give signals, direct or indirect, to indicate they are considering suicide because many people have some ambivalence and want help. Others may act impulsively or effectively hide their distress.

Euthanasia and Physician-Assisted Suicide

Euthanasia (mercy killing) is bringing about the death of someone deliberately and without legal standing in order to save them from suffering. This usually happens through the administration of high dose opioids although some people, usually family members, have resorted to more violent means, such as through gunshots or smothering. In some cases, euthanasia is carried out at the request of the patient, but it may be involuntary in other cases. Euthanasia is illegal in all states.

Physician-assisted suicide, on the other hand, requires that a patient be of sound mind and go through a legal process verifying that the patient's condition is terminal and the patient chooses to die. Physician-assisted suicide is legal in some form in California, Colorado, the District of Columbia, Hawaii, Maine, New Mexico, New Jersey, Oregon, Vermont, and Washington in the United States. In these states, physicians can order drugs that will bring about death.

Ethical Issues Related to Sedation of Hospice Palliative Care Patients

Palliative sedation (sometimes referred to as *terminal sedation*) is often used in the end-stages of dying to relieve severe pain and suffering. Patients usually receive analgesia along with a sedative so that they can die peacefully although they are no longer able to communicate with family members, so there is a tradeoff. There is concern among some people, especially those opposed to physician-assisted suicide, that sedation may hasten death and is, in fact, a method of slow euthanasia. However, most patients at this time are also unable to take food or fluids, and studies have shown that the addition of sedation does not hasten death and, in fact, may prolong life because the stress and exhaustion of experiencing severe pain or dyspnea is relieved. One concern is that there is no standard guideline for this type of sedation and practices vary.

Patients' Rights

The rights of patients and their families in relation to what they should expect from a healthcare organization are outlined in standards of both the Joint Commission and the National Committee for Quality Assurance. Rights include:

- Respect for the patient, including personal dignity and psychosocial, spiritual, and cultural considerations
- Response to needs related to access and pain control
- Ability to make decisions about care, including informed consent, advance directives, and end of life care
- Procedure for registering complaints or grievances
- Protection of confidentiality and privacy
- Freedom from abuse or neglect

- Protection during research and information related to ethical issues of research
- Appraisal of outcomes, including unexpected outcomes
- Information about organization, services, and practitioners
- Appeal procedures for decisions regarding benefits and quality of care
- Organizational code of ethical behavior
- Procedures for donating and procuring organs/tissue

CONFIDENTIALITY

Confidentiality is the obligation that is present in a professional-patient relationship. Nurses are under an obligation to protect the information they possess concerning the patient and family. Care should be taken to safeguard that information and provide the privacy that the patient deserves. This is accomplished through the use of required passwords when family call for information about the patient and through the limitation of who is allowed to visit. The nurse should not assume that family members can be apprised of an older adult's health information without that person's consent. There may be times when confidentiality must be broken to save the life of a patient or others, but those circumstances are rare. The nurse must make all efforts to safeguard patient records and identification. Computerized record keeping should be done in such a way that the screen is not visible to others, and paper records must be secured.

HIPAA

HIPAA regulations are designed to protect the rights of individuals regarding the privacy of their health information. The nurse must not release any information or documentation about an individual's condition or treatment without consent, as the individual has the right to determine who has access to personal information. Personal information about the individual is considered **protected health information (PHI)**, and consists of any identifying or personal information about the individual, such as health history, condition, or treatments in any form, and any documentation, including electronic, verbal, or written. Personal information can be shared with the spouse, legal guardians, those with durable power of attorney for the individual, and those involved in care of the individual, such as physicians, without a specific release, but the individual should always be consulted if personal information is to be discussed with others present to ensure there is no objection. Failure to comply with HIPAA regulations can make a nurse liable for legal action.

Review Video: HIPAA
Visit mometrix.com/academy and enter code: 412009

ADVANCE DIRECTIVES, DNR, AND DURABLE POWER OF ATTORNEY

In accordance to Federal and state laws, individuals have the right to self-determination in health care, including decisions about end-of-life care through **advance directives** such as living wills and the right to assign a surrogate person to make decisions through a **durable power of attorney**. Patients should routinely be questioned about an advanced directive as they may present at a healthcare organization without the document. Patients who have indicated they desire a **do-not-resuscitate (DNR)** order should not receive resuscitative treatments for terminal illness or conditions in which meaningful recovery cannot occur. Patients and families of those with terminal illnesses should be questioned as to whether the patients are hospice patients. For those with DNR requests or those withdrawing life support, staff should provide the patient palliative rather than curative measures, such as pain control and oxygen, and emotional support to the patient and family. Religious traditions and beliefs about death should be treated with respect.

Scope of Practice

Nurse Practice Act

Each state has its own Nurse Practice Act, which is administered by the state Board of Nursing. The Nurse Practice Act outlines requirements for licensure and certification and delineates the scope of practice of nurses, including duties and delegation. Typically, licensure is granted to those who complete an accredited LVN/LPN or RN program and pass the nursing exam (NCLEX) or receive endorsement because of licensure in another state. RN programs may be 3-year hospital-based programs, associate degree programs, or bachelor's degree programs. Foreign-trained nurses may need to meet special requirements that are determined by the state Board of Nursing and included in the Nurse Practice Act. Advance practice nurses complete a master's or doctorate program. The Nurse Practice Act of each state provides the requirement for advanced practice certification and the professional designation. Additionally, the Nurse Practice Act outlines the requirements for relicensing or recertification, often including the need for continuing education. The Nurse Practice Act also includes provisions for disciplinary action.

Incorporating National Standards into Nursing Practice

Incorporating national hospital and palliative standards into nursing practice includes:

- Obtaining a commitment from administration and staff members
- Researching and identifying appropriate national standards and practice guidelines to apply to practice, such as those of the National Consensus Project
- Assessing current status to identify gaps in practice, such as through gap analysis
- Educating staff members about the standards and changes in practice needed to meet standards
- Establishing a timeline for training and implementation of practice guidelines to achieve standards
- Providing ongoing in-service training to ensure that standards are instituted properly and that staff members have necessary knowledge and skills
- Determining appropriate measurement tools to assess progress
- Conducting ongoing measures to evaluate implementation and outcomes
- Reviewing outcome measures to determine if gaps still remain
- Providing progress reports to administration and staff on a regular basis

National Consensus Project Guidelines

Major hospice and palliative care organizations have joined forces to form the **National Consensus Project**:

- American Academy of Hospice and Palliative Medicine
- Center to Advance Palliative Care
- Hospice and Palliative Nurses Association
- National Hospice and Palliative Care Organization
- Partnership for Caring: America's Voice for the Dying

The National Consensus Project published 8 clinical practice guidelines that outlined standards for palliative care, most recently updated in 2018. Practice **guidelines** include:

- Structure and Processes of Care
- Physical Aspects of Care
- Psychological and Psychiatric Aspects of Care
- Social Aspects of Care
- Spiritual, Religious, and Existential Aspects of Care
- Cultural Aspects of Care
- Care of the Patient Nearing the End of Life
- Ethical and Legal Aspects of Care

Each practice guideline contains a number of sub-guidelines with criteria for achieving that standard of care. For example, Structure and Processes of Care comprises 10 guidelines, such as Guideline 1.1 "Interdisciplinary Team."

National Hospice and Palliative Care Standards and Guidelines

Overview of Scope of Practice of ACHPN

The **advanced certified hospice and palliative nurse (ACHPN)** must practice within the standards of advance practice and the individual's scope of practice, which is directly related to the individual's educational preparation and certification. The ACHPN must be practicing as a clinical nurse specialist (CNS) or nurse practitioner (NP) and must have two types of licenses/certificates: an RN and an advanced practice certificate. Advance practice nurses are those who have completed additional education in an accredited nursing program (usually at a Master's level) and have received certification with a national certifying organization, such as the American Nurse's Credentialing Center. The ACHPN must function legally under the nurse practice act of the state in which the person resides. In some cases, a license/certification in one state is automatically recognized in other states through the Compact agreement, but advance practice nurses are often excluded from these agreements. Educational experience and scope of practice must relate to patient population in terms of age, disease, diagnosis, and treatment.

Scope and Standards of Advanced Practice

The ACHPN is guided by the **standards of advanced practice**, which provide the framework for practice and describes the ACHPN's responsibilities, related to the values and priorities of the profession:

- **Care process**: Assessing, diagnosing, developing, and implementing a plan of care, and evaluating the patient's response
- **Priorities**: Providing education and encouraging the patient/family to take an active role in self-care
- **Collaboration**: Consulting with others when appropriate and referring the patient to specialists as needed
- **Documentation**: Keeping accurate, legal, legible records and maintaining patient confidentiality
- **Patient advocacy**: Advocating for the individual patient in the process of care but also for patients at the state and national level in order to facilitate patient access to care and improve the quality of care
- **Continuous quality improvement**: Recognizing the need for constant learning, evaluation, and reevaluation and participating in quality review, continuing education while maintaining certification and utilizing clinical guidelines and standards of care
- **Research and education**: Initiating, participating in, and utilizing the results of research in clinical practice

Review Video: Patient Advocacy
Visit mometrix.com/academy and enter code: 202160

Services Covered by Scope of and Standards of Practice for ACHPN

As part of the scope of practice as an advanced practice nurse, the ACHPN is able to provide and augment care to hospice and palliative patients through various services:

- **Consultation**: Assessing risk factors, providing interventions (such as pain control, skin care, and nutritional assistance), and educating patients and families
- **Referral**: Referring to appropriate healthcare providers and to organizations or agencies, such as pharmaceutical assistance programs
- **Coordination**: Maintaining contact and receiving reports from referrals in order to provide an integrated plan of care, preventing duplication of services, and ensuring that issues are not overlooked
- **Prescription**: Furnishing/prescribing medications within state guidelines, maintaining a list of medications, and considering cost-effectiveness
- **Diagnostics**: Ordering EKGs and radiographic tests for routine screening and health assessment as well as diagnosis based on assessment

Self-Care

Stress Management Strategies

While it's not possible to eliminate all stress, nurses can learn to manage stress so it has less emotional and physical impact on their lives. **Stress management strategies** include:

- **Meditation/breathing exercises**: Slow in and out while repeating a word or phrase
- **Massage**: Self-massage or by others
- **Progressive relaxation techniques**
- **Visualization/positive thinking**: Use the power of the mind to imagine a more positive outcome.
- **Time management**: Establish priorities, make schedule, and delegate.
- **Exercise**: Increase activity and exercise 20-30 minutes daily.
- **Breaks**: Plan regular breaks from work or other activities, 5-15 minutes.
- **Snacks**: Prepare healthy snacks and avoid high sugar/high fat snack foods.
- **Hobbies or interests**: Find an outlet, such as reading, music, painting, or crafts.

Critical Incident Stress Management

Critical incident stress management (CISM) is a procedure to help people cope with stressful events, such as disasters, in order to reduce incidence of post-traumatic stress syndrome. CISM can also help the hospice and palliative care staff members cope with the stress of caring for dying patients:

- **Defusing sessions** usually occur very early, sometimes during or immediately after a stressful event, and are used to educate personnel who are actively involved about what to expect over the next few days and to provide guidance in handling feelings and stress.
- **Debriefing sessions** usually follow in one to three days and may be repeated periodically as needed. These sessions may include people who were directly involved as well as those indirectly involved. People are encouraged to express their feelings and emotions about the event. The six phases of debriefing include introduction, fact sharing, discussing feelings, describing symptoms, teaching, and reentry. Critiquing the event or attempting to place blame is not productive as part of the CISM process.
- **Follow-up** is done at the end of the process, usually after about week but this can vary.

Burnout

Burnout, a response to ongoing stress, is a pervasive problem in the nursing profession. Nurses often have excessive workloads and work long hours, often including unwanted overtime because of inadequate staffing. Nurses may feel that they have little control over their work and do not receive sufficient reward or support and feel that nurses are often treated unfairly or are victims of bullying in the workplace. Stress tends to build up over time, interfering with the nurse's ability to concentrate and to carry out duties effectively. Burnout is one of the leading causes for nurses abandoning the field of nursing for other occupations. **Stages leading to burnout** include:

- Fight or flight response: Withdrawal, discord
- Emotional reaction: Anger, shock, surprise
- Negative thinking: Despair, anger, depression, anxiety
- Physical reaction: Headaches, GI upset, backache
- No change in stressor or person: Increased stress
- Burnout: Extreme exhaustion

Assessment Tools for Stress and Burnout

The **Professional Quality of Life Scale (ProQOL)** consists of 30 statements about feelings, such as "I feel connected to others," and "I feel trapped by my job." Each item on the tool is scored as (1) never, (2) rarely, (3) sometimes, (4) often, and (5) very often. Ten questions assess satisfaction, 10, burnout, and 10 secondary traumatic stress. The ratings are totaled for each set of 10 questions and the level is assigned as low, average, or high depending on the score.

The **Life Stress Test** lists possible events, such as retirement (45 points), death of a close friend (37 points), and change in work hour (20 points), and assigns point values. The points for those that apply are totaled. Scores of 0 to 149 indicate low risk for developing stress-related illness; 150-299, medium risk; and 300 and greater, high risk.

The **Empath Test** has 25 statements, such as "You sense others' pain and sadness" and "You feel drained around certain people." Each statement is scored as (0) never, (2), sometimes, or (3) always and the scores totaled. Score of 25-50 is that of a true empath.

Compassion Fatigue in Nurses

Compassion fatigue can occur when people overly identify with the pain and suffering of others and begin to exhibit signs of stress as a result. These people are often empathetic, tend to place the needs of others above their own, and are motivated by the need to help others. **Indications of compassion fatigue** include:

- Blaming others and complaining excessively
- Isolating oneself from others and having trouble concentrating
- Exhibiting compulsive activities (gambling, drinking)
- Having nightmares, sleeping poorly, and exhibiting a change in appetite
- Exhibiting sadness and/or apathy
- Denying any problems and having high expectations of self and others
- Having trouble concentrating
- Questioning spiritual beliefs, losing faith
- Exhibiting stress disorders: tachycardia, headaches, insomnia, pain

Healthcare providers who exhibit compassion fatigue may need to take a break from work in order to recover some sense of self and may benefit from stress management programs, cognitive behavioral therapy, relaxation and visualization exercises, and physical exercise.

Professional Communication and Clinical Decision-Making

Professional Communication Strategies

Communication strategies may involve verbal, nonverbal, and visual communication, depending on the situation. **Communication strategies** include:

- **Intrapersonal**: Dialog with the self is used in decision-making and aids in comprehension of input, planning for output, and personal assessment.
- **Interpersonal**: Face-to-face communication with others may be direct or electronic. Face-to-face communication facilitates all forms of communication, so many different types of communication may occur simultaneously, increasing the chance of the message being correctly received and persuading others.
- **Small group**: Small groups (3-6 individuals) allow a number of different relationships to develop and facilitate communication; however, if the group is too large, cliques may form. Members may be influenced positively or negatively by others, depending on the degree of cohesiveness.
- **Organizational**: May include intrapersonal, interpersonal, small group, and public communication, depending on the purpose of communication. Communication is often based on the hierarchical structure.
- **Public**: Information shared from the individual to a large group to inform, persuade, or entertain.

Eliciting Questions and Input from Others

The most important factor in **eliciting questions** and input from others is to remain attentive to what people are saying and how they are reacting because both provide opportunities for explorations of ideas and questioning. Restating comments or asking for clarification can encourage elaboration. Asking open-ended questions (who, what, when, why, where, how) results in a more detailed response than simple yes-or-no questions. It's important to always acknowledge and respond to patients' and families' comments and questions in an honest and forthright manner, showing respect for their ideas to encourage further exchange. The nurse can elicit questions and input from team members by asking for help reaching decisions or for information related to the person's area of expertise. The nurse should make a point of acknowledging others' contributions and providing positive feedback.

Utilizing Appropriate Team Members and Consultants

Team members and consultants have vital roles in meeting the needs of the patient:

- **Pharmacists**: Provide guidance on medications, especially analgesia and antiemetics, including interactions and adverse effects as well as dosage and equianalgesia.
- **Occupational therapists**: Can assist patients to compensate for physical weakness or deficits in order to allow them to remain independent in ADLs as long as possible.
- **Physical therapists**: Can help patients to maintain muscle strength and mobility and can recommend appropriate assistive devices.
- **Nutritionists**: Can provide nutritional guidance and assist the patient and family in finding foods that the patient can tolerate that do not exacerbate symptoms, such as nausea.
- **Spiritual advisor**: Can provide emotional support and help relieve anxiety as well as helping the patient and family members communicate more effectively.
- **Psychologist**: Can provide patients with tools to help deal with anxiety, depression, and other responses to disease.

Barriers to Effective Workplace Communication

Barriers to effective workplace communication include:

- **Psychological factors**: The emotional status of those communicating, such as increased anxiety, can negatively impact communication. Biases, prejudices, and belief systems may also interfere with a person's ability to attend to the ideas of another person.
- **Physical factors**: Communication may be impaired if there is excessive noise or distracting activities taking place. Some environments are not conducive to communication, especially if too great a distance separates the communicators.
- **Gender factors**: Communication styles often vary between males and females, and this can lead to misunderstanding. However, communication styles may also vary among those of the same gender depending on many social and psychological factors.
- **Semantic factors**: Communicators may have different understanding of the same words. For example, a speaker of English as a second language may have a more literal interpretation of words than a native speaker, which can lead to misunderstanding.

Conflict Management

Positive and Negative Effects of Conflict

Some type of **conflict** is usually inevitable in any group of individuals, and it should be viewed as an opportunity for reflection rather than a failing. In fact, there are both negative and positive effects of conflict:

- **Negative**: Conflict can result in impaired communication and resentment and can damage the cohesiveness of a group of individuals, especially if people begin to take sides. Heated disagreements can escalate to fighting and aggressive behavior, which can hinder performance.
- **Positive**: Conflict can result in new ideas and improved decision-making. Conflict can also result in increased creativity as individuals search for answers to the conflict and may bring about awareness for a need for better communication. Conflict can also result in increased interest and can provide a means of release of tension.

Conflict is best dealt with openly because unresolved conflicts can begin to mushroom into serious problems.

Primary Levels of Conflict

There are two primary **levels of conflict**:

- **Intrapersonal**: This type of conflict occurs within the individual, often when there are two competing needs or unmet needs. This can occur if a nurse is unhappy with an assignment or feels unable to provide the type of care desired because of job restrictions or inadequate staffing. This can manifest as withdrawal or anger.
- **Interpersonal**: This type of conflict occurs between or among individuals or groups. A typical example is a disagreement between a nurse and a doctor or between two nurses over issues of patient care or personal matters. Subtypes of interpersonal conflict include intragroup, intergroup, and interorganizational conflicts, such as disagreements between two departments and between nurses and doctors. A group may be splintered by different opinions. Intergroup and interorganizational conflict may be difficult to resolve, especially if many people are involved, because of competing interests, and may require mediation.

Primary Types of Conflict

The three primary **types of conflict** include:

- **Relationship**: This is characterized by interpersonal conflicts that revolve around personal feelings and discord, such as a disagreement between two individuals. When relationship conflict is present, this can have a profoundly negative effect on team satisfaction and function, especially because people tend to become polarized, supporting one position or the other.
- **Task**: This is characterized by differences of opinions in how to accomplish a task, and it can result in heated discussions, but it rarely degenerates into negativity in the same way that relationship conflict does. Resolution should be evidence-based as much as possible.
- **Process**: This is characterized by differences of opinion about who is responsible for accomplishing a task. For example, group members may disagree about who is responsible for ordering supplies. This type of conflict is usually the easiest to resolve by compromise.

Conflict Resolution

Conflict is an almost inevitable product of teamwork, and the nurse must assume responsibility for conflict resolution. While conflicts can be disruptive, they can produce positive outcomes by forcing team members to listen to different perspectives and opening dialogue. The team should make a plan for dealing with conflict resolution. The best time for conflict resolution is when differences emerge but before open conflict and hardening of positions occur. The leader must pay close attention to the people and problems involved, listen carefully, and reassure those involved that their points of view are understood. Steps to **conflict resolution** include:

- Allow both sides to present their side of conflict without bias, maintaining a focus on opinions rather than individuals.
- Encourage cooperation through negotiation and compromise.
- Maintain the focus, providing guidance to keep the discussions on track and avoid arguments.
- Evaluate the need for renegotiation, formal resolution process, or third party.
- Utilize humor and empathy to diffuse escalating tensions.
- Summarize the issues, outlining key arguments.
- Avoid forcing resolution if possible.

Professional Documentation

Overview

Documentation is a form of communication that provides information about the healthcare individual and confirms that care was provided. Accurate, objective, and complete documentation of individual care is required by both accreditation and reimbursement agencies, including federal and state governments. **Purposes** of documentation include:

- Carrying out professional responsibility.
- Establishing accountability.
- Communicating among health professionals.
- Educating staff.
- Providing information for research.
- Satisfying legal and practice standards.
- Ensuring reimbursement.

While documentation focuses on progress notes, there are many other aspects to charting. Doctor's orders must be noted, medication administration must be documented on medication sheets, and vital signs must be graphed. Flow sheets must be checked off, filled out, or initialed. Admission assessments may involve primarily checklists or may require extensive documentation. The primary issue in malpractice cases is inaccurate or incomplete documentation. It's better to over-document than under, but effective documentation does neither.

Accuracy

Regardless of format, documentation should always include any change in a patient's condition, any treatments, medications, or other interventions, patient responses, and any complaints from the family or patient. Nurses should avoid subjective descriptions (especially negative terms, which could be used to establish bias in court), such as tired, angry, confused, bored, rude, happy, and euphoric. Instead, more objective descriptions ("Yawning 2-3 times a minute") should be used. Patients can be quoted directly ("I shouldn't have to wait for medication when I need it"). Charting should focus on nursing diagnoses. Nurses should chart every 1-2 hours for routine care (bathing, walking), but medications and other interventions or changes in condition should be charted immediately. A standardized vocabulary should be used for documenting, including lists of approved abbreviations and symbols. Abbreviations and symbols especially can pose serious problems in interpretation, so they should be used sparingly.

Interdisciplinary Collaboration

Interdisciplinary collaboration is absolutely critical to nursing practice in order to develop collaborative agreements and practice protocols. Collaborative practice agreements are formal relationships, most often between a physician and an advanced practice nurse that includes guidelines for collaboration, consultation, and referral. Interdisciplinary practice begins with the nurse and physician but extends to pharmacists, social workers, occupational and physical therapists, nutritionists, and a wide range of allied healthcare providers, all of whom cooperate in diagnosis, treatment, and planning. While advanced practice nurses have increasingly gained more legal rights, they have also become more dependent upon collaboration with others for their expertise and for referrals if the individual's needs extend beyond the nurse's ability to provide assistance or to plan for care.

Methods of Promoting Collaboration

Promoting collaboration and assisting others to understand and use the resources and expertise of others require a commitment in terms of time and effort:

- **Coaching** others on methods of collaboration can include providing information in the form of handouts about effective communication strategies and modeling this type of communication with the staff being coached.
- **Team meetings** are commonly held on nursing units, and they provide an opportunity to model collaboration and suggest the need for outside expertise to help with patient care plans. The mentoring nurse can initiate discussions about resources that are available in the facility or the community.
- **Selecting a diverse group for teams** or inviting those with expertise in various areas to join the team when needed can help team members to appreciate and understand how to use the input of other resources.

Internal and External Collaboration

Collaboration through interdisciplinary teams is very common in healthcare and is a form of internal collaboration intended to improve healthcare.

- **Internal collaboration** takes place within an organization or program and may be formal or informal. A typical form of collaboration occurs when, for example, a nurse discusses how best to meet a patient's needs with an occupational therapist, benefitting from the knowledge of another professional. Internal collaboration is often face-to-face but may also be carried out by phone, text message, or email, especially in large organizations where opportunities for face-to-face meetings are limited.
- **External collaboration** is often more formal and involves collaboration with those outside the organization often brought about by alliances, partnerships, and joint ventures. External collaboration may be motivated by the need for expertise not available in-house. External collaboration can be facilitated by technology, such as video conferencing.

Interpersonal Communication Skills Needed for Collaboration

Collaboration requires a number of interpersonal communication skills that differ from those involved in communication between nurse and individual. These skills include:

- **Using an assertive approach**: It's important for the nurse to honestly express opinions and to state them clearly and with confidence, but the nurse must do so in a calm non-threatening manner.
- **Making casual conversation**: It's easier to communicate with people with whom one has a personal connection. Asking open-ended questions, asking about another person's work, or commenting on someone's contributions helps to establish a relationship. The time before meetings, during breaks, and after meetings presents an opportunity for this type of conversation.
- **Being competent in public speaking**: Collaboration requires that a nurse be comfortable speaking and presenting ideas to groups of people. Doing so helps a person gain credibility. This is a skill that must be practiced.
- **Communicating in writing**: The written word remains a critical component of communication, and the nurse should be able to communicate clearly and grammatically.

Teamwork

Teambuilding

Leading, facilitating, and participating in performance improvement teams requires a thorough understanding of the dynamics of **teambuilding**:

- **Initial interactions**: This is the time when members begin to define their roles and develop relationships, determining if they are comfortable in the group.
- **Power issues**: The members observe the leader and determine who controls the meeting and how control is exercised, beginning to form alliances.
- **Organizing**: Methods to achieve work are clarified and team members begin to work together, gaining respect for each other's contributions and working toward a common goal.
- **Team identification**: Interactions often become less formal as members develop rapport, and members are more willing to help and support each other to achieve goals.
- **Excellence**: This develops through a combination of good leadership, committed team members, clear goals, high standards, external recognition, a spirit of collaboration, and a shared commitment to the process.

Team Structure

The appropriate team structure is very important in performance improvement because creating a team does not in itself assure teamwork. The team must be comprised of individuals whose skills complement each other and who have a shared purpose because outcomes will depend on the collaborative efforts of the group rather than individuals within the group. Accordingly, the collective team is accountable for outcomes rather than individuals. When creating teams, important elements that affect the **team structure** must be considered:

- **Size**: Teams of <10 members are most effective.
- **Skills**: Team members should have complementary skills that encompass technical, problem solving, decision making, and interpersonal.
- **Performance goals**: Teams should be allowed a degree of autonomy in producing action plans for performance improvement, based on strategic goals and objectives.
- **Unified approach**: The teams should be created according to the model of performance improvement, but should have some flexibility in working together.
- **Accountability**: The team members are collectively accountable rather than individually.

Self-Directed Work Teams

Self-directed work teams are groups of individuals working together to achieve a common goal, such as improving a process or producing a product. While the members may be trained cross-functionally, they usually have individual functions within the group. Usually, the teams have an assigned task or tasks for which they are accountable and have the authority to manage the functions on their own and make decisions without the direction of administration. As with other types of teams, self-directed work teams may be *ad hoc* or permanent and the degree of autonomy may vary from one organization to another. **Self-directed work teams** may do the following:

- Plan and establish priorities
- Organize and manage budget
- Manage work schedules and assignments
- Engage in problem-solving activities and make corrections
- Monitor and evaluate performance
- Coordinate with other teams or individuals
- Chose or hire team members

Coordination of Intra- and Interdisciplinary Teams

There are a number of skills that are needed to lead and facilitate coordination of intra- and interdisciplinary teams:

- Communicating openly is essential with all members encouraged to participate as valued members of a cooperative team.
- Avoiding interrupting or interpreting the point another is trying to make allows free flow of ideas.
- Avoiding jumping to conclusions, which can effectively shut off communication.
- Active listening requires paying attention and asking questions for clarification rather than to challenge others' ideas.
- Respecting others' opinions and ideas, even when opposed to one's own, is absolutely essential.
- Reacting and responding to facts rather than feelings allows one to avoid angry confrontations or diffuse anger.

- Clarifying information or opinions stated can help avoid misunderstandings.
- Keeping unsolicited advice out of the conversation shows respect for others and allows them to solicit advice without feeling pressured.

Continuous Quality Improvement

Performance Improvement Models

A number of different performance improvement models have been developed over the years. Evaluating and applying these models are part of strategic management and quality healthcare. In some organizations, one approach may be used, but often models are combined in various ways in order to meet specific needs. Planning and understanding how these models can facilitate change are important for those in leadership roles because, in order for these models to be effective, there must be cooperation and consensus across the organization. The various models share some like elements:

- The models focus on continuous improvement and are planned, systematic, and collaborative and apply to the entire organization.
- They share a common focus on identifying problems, collecting data, assessing current performance, instituting actions for change, assessing changes, team development, and use of data.

A model or models should be chosen that seem appropriate to the needs of the organization and to those who will work with the model.

CQI

Continuous Quality Improvement (CQI) emphasizes the organization and systems and processes within that organization rather than individuals. It recognizes internal customers (staff) and external customers (patients) and utilizes data to improve processes. CQI represents the concept that most processes can be improved. CQI uses the scientific method of experimentation to meet needs and improve services and utilizes various tools, such as brainstorming, multivoting, various charts and diagrams, storyboarding, and meetings. Core concepts include:

- Reaching quality and success is meeting or exceeding internal and external customer's needs and expectations.
- Problems relate to processes, and variations in process lead to variations in results.
- Change can be in small steps.

Steps to CQI include:

- Form a knowledgeable team.
- Identify and defining measures used to determine success.
- Brainstorm strategies for change.
- Plan, collect, and utilize data as part of making decisions.
- Test changes and revise or refine as needed.

PDCA Method of Quality Improvement

Plan-Do-Check-Act (PDCA) is a method of continuous quality improvement. PDCA is simple and understandable; however, it may be difficult to maintain this cycle consistently because of lack of focus and commitment. PDCA may be more suited to solving specific problems than organization-wide problems:

- **Plan**: Identifying, analyzing, and defining the problem, clearly defining it setting goals, and establishing a process that coordinates with leadership. Extensive brainstorming, including fishbone diagrams, identifies problematic processes and lists current process steps. Data is collected and analyzed and root cause analysis completed.
- **Do**: Generating possible solutions from which to select one or more and then implementing the solution on a trial basis.
- **Check**: Gathering and analyzing data to determine the effectiveness of the solution. If effective, then continue to Act; if not, return to Plan and pick a different solution. (*Study* may sometimes be used in place of *Check*: PDSA.)
- **Act**: Identifying changes that need to be done to fully implement solution, adopting the solution, and continuing to monitor results while picking another improvement project.

Gap Analysis

Gap analysis is a method used to determine the steps required to move from a current state or actual performance or situation to a new state or potential performance or situation and the "gap" between the two that requires action or resources. Essentially gap analysis answers the questions "What is our current situation?" and "What do we want it to become?" Gap analysis includes determining the resources and time required to achieve the target goal. **Steps to gap analysis** include:

- Assessing the current situation and listing important factors, such as performance levels, costs, staffing, satisfaction, and all processes
- Identifying the current outcomes of the processes in place
- Identifying the target outcomes for projected processes
- Outlining the process required to achieve target outcomes
- Identifying the gaps that are present between the current process and goal
- Identifying resources and methods to close the gaps

TQM

Total Quality Management (TQM) is one philosophy of quality management that espouses a commitment to meeting the needs of the customers at all levels within an organization. It promotes not only continuous improvement but also a dedication to quality in all aspects of an organization. Outcomes should include increased customer satisfaction and productivity, as well as increased profits through efficiency and reduction in costs. In order to provide TQM, an organization must seek the following:

- Information regarding customer's needs and opinions.
- Involvement of staff at all levels in decision making, goal setting, and problem solving.
- Commitment of management to empowering staff and being accountable through active leadership and participation.
- Institution of teamwork with incentives and rewards for accomplishments.

The focus of TQM is on working together to identify and solve problems rather than assigning blame through an organizational culture that focuses on the needs of the customers.

Hospice Criteria

Advocating for Hospice and Palliative Care

The nurse can advocate for hospice and palliative care by:

- Joining professional organizations and participating in activities
- Writing articles (journals, newspapers, magazines) regarding hospice and palliative care
- Speaking in public forums (community meetings, social gatherings) about the importance of hospice and palliative care
- Utilizing social media
- Mentoring and coaching other nurses to help them become proficient in hospice and palliative care
- Completing continuing education courses in the field in order to remain current
- Discussing the role of nurses in hospice and palliative care with physicians
- Addressing administration and the board of directors regarding patient care and professional needs
- Developing training courses for other staff members
- Participating in development of community information resources, such as pamphlets
- Representing the profession in an ethical manner

Barriers across Health Care Settings

Barriers across health care settings include:

- **Geographic**: Some areas, especially rural, lack adequate healthcare resources, such as hospice and palliative care programs, hospitals, clinics, and physicians. Providing services is often not cost-effective for organizations.
- **Financial/insurance**: Many people lack financial resources to pay for adequate insurance coverage and cannot afford out-of-pocket payment for services.
- **Transportation**: People who do not have motor vehicles or no longer drive are at a disadvantage in accessing health care. Public transportation is not available in many areas and can be expensive for those on limited income.
- **Education/health literacy**: People with limited education or those who are functionally illiterate may lack the health literacy needed to understand their health needs or the healthcare services that are available.
- **Fear/anxiety**: People may fear medical care itself or fear hearing bad news, but both types of fears can prevent people from accessing the medical care that they need.

Initiating, Developing, and Fostering Hospice and Palliative Care Services

Strategies to initiate, develop, and foster hospice and palliative care services include:

- Providing continuing education credit for palliative care and hospice training sessions
- Visiting physicians, nurse practitioners, hospitals, and other health care providers and organizations to disseminate information
- Hosting an open-house or other event to publicize the services
- Budgeting for marketing expenses
- Tracking results of marketing activities
- Emphasizing collaboration and partnerships with other healthcare organizations
- Publishing a newsletter for healthcare professionals and community members
- Placing ads and/or public service announcements in local newspapers, television, and radio

- Sponsoring conferences regarding palliative and hospice care
- Reviewing potential barriers
- Providing excellence in patient care and services
- Serving as a referral source
- Utilizing social media in a responsible manner to market services

Application of Business Strategies to Hospice and Palliative Care

Organizations that provide hospice and palliative care often benefit from application of **business strategies**:

- **Internal review**: Determine what unique characteristics the organization has that can provide an advantage over other organizations. This includes measurements across all aspects of the organization to determine current status in relation to other organizations.
- **External review**: Assess community needs and determining where deficits occur to identify opportunities for provision of additional services. Determine the organization's market and resources as well as any obstacles the organization faces.
- **Growth initiatives**: Planning should look at opportunities for expansion, addition of staff, and addition of services.
- **Cost-benefit analysis**: Services, supplies, and equipment should be assessed in terms of return on investment, and cost-cutting measures taken where they do not impact the quality of service, such as buying in bulk and using different vendors.
- **Planning**: The organization should develop a comprehensive plan for the future and the direction the organization wants to take.

Application of Market Analysis to Hospice and Palliative Care

Market analysis is done to determine both the current status of the market for a product or service and the future potential. Market analysis includes assessment of the following:

- **Size of the market and demand**: Current data about sales from government, industry, surveys, and major producers of similar products or services
- **Marketing trends**: Regulations, social factors, environmental factors, innovations, and any factors that may affect sales
- **Growth rate of market**: Based on analysis of historical data and current sales data as well as developments that may impact growth positively or negatively
- **Opportunity assessment**: In terms of competition
- **Profitability**: Assessment of influencing factors (Porter), including buyer and supplier power, barriers to market entry, possible threat of competitive substitute products/services, and company rivalry
- **Cost structure**: Determining value and costs
- **Methods of distribution**: Existing and emerging
- **Necessary factors**: Resources, access to distribution, technology

Application of Maximized Reimbursement to Hospice and Palliative Care

Methods to maximize reimbursement include:

- Timely recording of information and sending of claims
- Utilizing care managers to determine the most cost-effective care plan
- Utilizing standardized billing codes (CPT, ICD)

- Ensuring that the healthcare provider's National Provider Identifier (NPI) is present on all claims
- Updating systems promptly when new coding (such as ICD-10) and billing regulations (such as pay-for-performance) are issued rather than waiting for the end of the grace period so that problems can be identified and corrected early
- Ensuring that the present on admission (POA) Medicare Severity-Diagnosis Related Group (MS-DRG) diagnosis is correct to avoid a different discharge diagnosis
- Monitoring quality of care to prevent complications and reduce costs related to the Do Not Pay List
- Sending claims in the correct form and to the correct address for different entities, such as insurance companies, Medicaid, or Medicare

Promoting Continuity of Care

Many forces disrupt the **continuity of care**. In some cases, physicians (or advanced care nurses) no longer follow patients from the home to the in-patient facility because care at each level is managed by different health care providers, such as hospitalists. While this has some advantages, patients are often cared for by healthcare providers who don't actually know them or their history, so the most important factor in promoting continuity of care is communication. Case managers and discharge planners are critical to improving continuity of care by ensuring that all parties understand patients' needs and that patients and families understand their rights and responsibilities. Healthcare providers must make sure that patients have signed appropriate releases of medical records so that information can be shared. Hospice and palliative care organizations need to establish partnerships and good working relationships with other providers of healthcare services.

Facilitating Safe Passage

Facilitating safe passage is part of caring practice that ensures patient safety, in a broad sense, from a variety of perspectives:

- Giving appropriate medications and treatment without errors that endanger the patient's health is essential.
- Providing information to the patient/family about treatments, changes, conditions, and other aspects related to care helps them to cope with situations as they arise.
- Preventing infection is central to patient safety and includes staff using proper infection control methods, such as handwashing.
- Knowing the person requires the nurse to take the time and effort to understand the needs and wishes of the patient/family.
- Assisting with transitions involves not only helping the patient/family cope with moving from one form of treatment, or one unit to another but also with transitions in health, such as from health to illness, or from illness to death.

Health Insurance Options

Types and Characteristics of Health Insurance

Types and characteristics of health insurance include:

- **HMO**: With health maintenance organizations (HMOs), a primary care provider (PCP) coordinates care and referrals to a network of healthcare providers. The individual has little choice and requires a referral from the PCP to see a specialist. Plans may provide preventive care but may also require co-payments and a deductible.

- **PPO**: With a preferred provider organization (PPO) an individual can choose to see any healthcare provider, including specialists, in a network of healthcare providers. The individual is not usually required to select a PCP but may have to pay co-payments and a deductible, depending on the plan. Individuals can usually see healthcare providers outside of the network but reimbursement is typically lower, so the individual may have to pay part of costs.
- **EPO**: The exclusive provider organization (EPO) is similar to a PPO in that the individual can see any physician within a network except that the individual does not have the option of seeing a healthcare provider outside of the network except in emergency situations.
- **POS**: Point of service plans (POSs) are combined HMOs and PPOs. The individual has a PCP within a network, and the PCP makes referrals, but the individual can see out-of-network healthcare providers. The individual must pay part of cost to see out-of-network providers.
- **HDHP**: High deductible health plans (HDHPs) may be HMOs, PPOs, or EPOs but are characterized by a high deductible before the insurance begins to reimburse for care. People with low-income often select this option to avoid catastrophic costs but may end up with large bills for healthcare services.

Medicare

Medicare, a federal health insurance program for those who have Social Security or bought into Medicare, provides payment to private healthcare providers, such as physicians and hospitals, but limits reimbursement. Physicians receive 80% of usual customary and reasonable (UCR) fees if they accept Medicare assignment. If they do not, they can charge up to 115% of what Medicare allows. Patients are responsible for the remaining 20% or up to 115% if the physicians do not accept Medicare. Parts include:

- **Medicare A**: Hospital insurance covers acute hospital care, limited nursing home care, and home health care as well as hospice care for the terminally ill. There is no premium for this part.
- **Medicare B**: Medical insurance covers physicians, advance practice nurses, laboratory, physical and occupational therapy. Patients must pay an annual deductible as well as monthly payments.
- **Medicare D**: The prescription drug plan covers part of the costs of prescription drugs at participating pharmacies. It is administered by private insurance companies, so monthly costs and benefits vary somewhat.

Medicaid

Medicaid is a combined federal and state welfare program authorized by Title XIX of the Social Security Act to assist people with low income with payment for medical care. This program provides assistance for all ages, including children. Older adults receiving SSI are eligible as are others who meet state eligibility requirements. The Medicaid programs are administered by the individual states, which establish eligibility and reimbursement guidelines, so benefits vary considerably from one state to another. Older adults with Medicare are eligible for Medicaid as a secondary insurance. Expenses that are covered include inpatient and outpatient hospital services, physician payments, nursing home care, home health care, and laboratory and radiation services. Adults who are legal resident aliens are ineligible for Medicaid for 5 years after attaining legal resident status. Some states pay for preventive services, such as home and community-based programs aimed at reducing the need for hospitalization.

Tricare

Tricare is the health care program serving active military, retired military, and their spouses and dependents. Tricare provides a number of different plans, depending upon location and eligibility. For those with Medicare, Tricare becomes the secondary insurer. If patients choose to opt out of Medicare (such as those with no insurance or private insurance), Tricare pays the amount equivalent to a secondary insurer (20% of allowable), and the patient is responsible for the rest. By law, all other insurances must pay before Tricare. Patients may access care at military treatment facilities (MTF) on space-available basis, but must enroll in Tricare Plus to receive primary care at MTFs. Those eligible for both Tricare and Veterans Affairs (VA) programs may receive care at VA medical facilities if the service is covered under Tricare and the facility is part of the Tricare network. It is important to note, the VA cannot bill Medicare, so costs not covered by Tricare must be paid by the patient even if the patient has Medicare coverage.

Coverage for Hospice Care

While palliative care may be utilized during all stages of illness, **hospice care** is for the terminally ill, usually within the last 6 months of life (two 90-day periods) although this may be extended by physician authorization every 60 days. Medicare patients must be eligible for Medicare A, and a physician must certify that the patient is terminal with life expectancy ≤6 months. The patient (or responsible family member) must agree to receive Hospice care rather than regular Medicare, requiring that the patient receive palliative rather than curative treatment. The goal of hospice care is to maintain the person in the home environment, so the patient is provided home health aides and homemakers, durable goods (dressings, adult diapers, under pads), pain management, case management, counseling, and social worker assistance. Routine home care is intermittent and must comprise 80% of total care. In-home continuous care is available during crisis for short periods. In-patient hospice (often beds assigned in a skilled nursing facility) may be used for 4-5 days for symptom management and/or a 5-day respite period for caregivers.

Causes of Lapses in Health Care Coverage Related to Hospice and Palliative Care

Lapses in health care coverage related to hospice and palliative care most often result from lack of insurance or limitations of insurance:

- **High deductibles**: To save money on premiums, some people opt for insurance policies with high deductibles, resulting in thousands of dollars in costs before insurance coverage begins.
- **Lack of insurance**: Some people have no insurance because they are unable to afford it or simply choose to gamble that they won't need it, but they may end up with huge medical bills and may not be eligible for Medicaid assistance.
- **Home health care**: Patients may need care in the home but lack qualifying hospital stays for Medicare coverage or lack insurance for home health care.
- **Hospice benefits**: Patients may not qualify for hospice benefits because their life expectancy is greater than 6 months, they don't have Medicare coverage, or their insurance does not cover hospice care.

Cost of Drugs

The cost of drugs is one of the most expensive aspects of medical care for patient, so patients sometimes can't afford treatment. Even those with insurance drug coverage or Medicare D may have considerable costs, especially with non-generic drugs. There is much pressure from drug representatives to prescribe new drugs, and patients are often influenced by direct-to-consumer advertising, but the ACHPN can help the patient ensure that drugs are prescribed based on evidence. Additionally, the cost versus benefit of drugs must always be considered. It is the responsibility of the ACHPN to act in the best interests of the patient and to educate the patient about drugs. If a less expensive drug is as effective as a more expensive or newer drug, then the ACHPN and patient should request that the less expensive drug be prescribed. The ACHPN should educate people about the use of generic drugs as a cost-saving measure because, in most cases, these are as effective as non-generic.

Professional Development

Pertinent Nursing Activities

Hospice and palliative care is a changing field of medicine. **Nurse responsibilities** to ensure professional competence in hospice and palliative care include:

- **Maintaining licensure and certification**: Renewing license/certification and completing continuing education courses or other requirements
- **Remaining current in education**: Reading and studying current journal articles and texts regarding neuroscience, taking courses, carrying out literature reviews, evaluating sources and research, participating in evidence-based research, and considering application of findings to current practice
- **Serving as a mentor and coach**: Sharing expertise and helping others to improve their knowledge and skills
- Participating in **state and national organizations**, such as the National Hospice and Palliative Care Organization and the American Nurses Association
- **Collaborating with others**: Patient, family, and other healthcare providers
- **Communicating effectively**: In written, oral, and visual communication forms
- **Maintaining high ethical standards**: In all circumstances and reporting any lapses to the appropriate authorities

SMART Technique for Professional Plan Development

Career planning is an ongoing endeavor that includes self-evaluation and goal setting in order to determine what path the individual wants to take as part of a professional development plan. The individual should develop both a short-term and a long-term career plan, determining where the person wants to be at a point in the future, such as in 5 years. The individual should conduct a career search, including the job market for potential careers and costs of education. One way to determine goals and establish a plan is to utilize the **SMART technique**:

- **S**pecific: Identify concrete actions and desired results ("Employment as nursing instructor")
- **M**easurable: Describe assessment parameters ("Work full time in university program")
- **A**chievable: Appropriate for scope of practice and situation ("Studies show need for nursing instructors and opportunities for employment, and grants available for students")
- **R**elevant/Realistic: Opportunities exist ("Local universities advertising for nursing instructors")
- **T**ime-framed: Beginning and ending dates for meeting goals ("Achieve goal within 3 years")

Sharing Evidence-Based Knowledge

There are a number of ways to communicate **evidence-based knowledge** about procedures, products, patient care, or technology:

- Presentations to administration and those in positions of leadership, such as team leaders or managers, to garner support for incorporating findings into practice
- In-service training/education that focuses on results of research and explains applicability
- Print distribution in the form of flyers or newsletters that outlines findings
- Electronic newsletters or training modules that present information of interest
- Discussions with intra- and interdisciplinary team members about research and ways in which to apply research to the practice of care

Communicating is only one part of the process. Procedures must be in place in each organization that outline the steps to incorporating evidence-based findings into practice. An inter-disciplinary team should evaluate research findings and together create a system-wide approach to application, with the goal to improve outcomes for patients.

MENTORING

The nurse is in an ideal position to serve as a **mentor**, both informally and formally. There are a number of elements that enhance mentoring:

- **Nurturing**: Being supportive and interested in furthering the skills and education of the staff
- **Providing clinical expertise**: Guiding the staff by demonstrating a personal commitment to excellence in provision of care
- **Motivating others**: Encouraging others and supporting them throughout their careers
- **Providing an example**: Teaching others by being a good example
- **Listening**: Being non-judgmental in discussions with others and listening to determine different perspectives and needs
- **Providing feedback**: Being honest in evaluation and assisting others to improve care, providing feedback about how their practices affect patient outcomes
- **Role modeling**: Providing assistance to others in gaining certification and in understanding the role of the hospice and palliative care nurse

PRECEPTORING

The nurse is often in the position of having many roles in clinical practice, including educating others and serving as a **preceptor** for graduate students who are studying to enter the field. While mentoring may entail a long-term relationship, precepting is usually a time-limited arrangement related to a term of study, such as a semester, orientation period, or a clinical rotation. The nurse must balance responsibilities and ensure that he or she is able to provide adequate clinical supervision and guidance to the student on a daily basis. This may require coordinating schedules and planning carefully to ensure all responsibilities can be met. The nurse preceptor helps the student to understand his or her impact on the spheres of influence (patient/client, nurse and nurse practice, and organization/system) by including the student in all nursing activities. The preceptor may engage in shared care as well as direct supervision in order to improve the student's skills.

COACHING

Coaching is an important part of mentoring/preceptoring. Coaching can include specific training, providing career information, and confronting issues of concern. While patient safety is the primary consideration, coaching should be done in a manner that increases learner confidence and ability to self-monitor rather than in a punitive or critical manner. The nurse must develop confidence in his/her own ability to be assertive and confront issues directly in order to resolve conflicts and promote collaboration. Effective **methods of coaching** include:

- Giving positive feedback, stressing what the student is doing right
- Using questioning to help the student recognize problem areas
- Providing demonstrations and opportunities for question/answer periods
- Providing regular progress reports so the student understands areas of concern
- Assisting the student to establish personal goals for improvement
- Providing resources to help the student master material

Developing Initiatives and Standards

An initiative is an introductory step or act that often involves developing standards. A standard provides a model that others should follow to obtain consistent results. Standards and initiatives should be designed so that they could remain current for a number of years. The process for **developing initiatives and standards** includes:

- Determine the need through assessment.
- Identify a sponsor to support development.
- Make a formal request.
- Develop a team or working group.
- Research best practices and evidence-based findings, carry out clinical research when appropriate.
- Draft a standard/initiative.
- Present the standard/initiative for comments.
- Allow appeals.
- Modify and/or correct the standard/initiative.
- Submit the initiative/standard to the appropriate body (administration, shared governance council, board of directors) for approval.
- Publish and distribute standard in various formats (print, PDF).
- Implement standard, measure results, obtain feedback.

ACHPN Practice Test

Want to take this practice test in an online interactive format?
Check out the online resources page, which includes interactive practice questions and much more: **mometrix.com/resources719/achpn**

1. A patient complains of inability to sleep because of persistent severe restless legs syndrome. Which of the following medications is most indicated?

a. Pramipexole.
b. Levo-dopa.
c. Cabergoline.
d. Gabapentin.

2. According to staging of tissue damage resulting from radiation, if the area is painful because of exposed nerves and the skin is moist and blistering with epidermal tissue having sloughed off and serous drainage is present, the damage would be classified as

a. stage I.
b. stage II.
c. stage III.
d. stage IV.

3. A COPD patient on corticosteroids has friable skin and has developed a skin tear with complete loss of tissue. This would be categorized according to the International Skin Tear Advisory Panel (ISTAP) Skin Tear Classification as

a. type 1.
b. type 2.
c. type 3.
d. type 4.

4. The factor that most indicates a risk of drug abuse or misuse after beginning chronic opioid therapy is

a. severe pain.
b. older age
c. preexisting cognitive impairment.
d. personal/family history of substance abuse.

5. For which of the following diagnoses may a patient be eligible for hospice care on diagnosis if the patient chooses to forego treatment?

a. Leukemia.
b. Small cell lung cancer.
c. Amyotrophic lateral sclerosis.
d. Multiple myeloma.

6. An 80-year-old non-diabetic patient with renal failure who has refused hemodialysis and is not a candidate for kidney transplantation has requested hospice services. Which of the following laboratory findings supports admission to hospice?

a. Creatinine clearance <10 mL/min and serum creatinine >8.0 mg/dL.
d. Creatinine clearance <10 mL/min and serum creatinine >4 mg/dL.
b. Creatinine clearance <15 mL/min and serum creatinine >7.0 mg/dL.
c. Creatinine clearance <15 mL/min and serum creatinine >6.0 mg/dL.

7. A patient with AIDS has a CD4+ count of 24, a viral load of 110,000, and a 35% drop in lean body mass. The Karnofsky Performance Scale score needed to qualify the patient for hospice care is

a. <70.
b. <60.
c. <50.
d. <40.

8. When the advanced practice registered nurse stays with a patient and holds the patient's hand when the physician delivers bad news about the patient's prognosis, the APRN is acting on the ethical principle of

a. nonmaleficence.
b. beneficence.
c. autonomy.
d. veracity.

9. If the advanced practice registered nurse is using the Palliative Performance Scale (PPS) to assess a patient with severe heart disease and finds the patient is now completely bedridden, requires total care, oral intake of both food and fluids is reduced, and the patient is responsive but very drowsy, the PPS score would be

a. 60.
b. 50.
c. 40.
d. 30.

10. A 46-year-old male with HIV/AIDS has anorexia and marked weight loss. Which of the following drugs may be indicated to relieve nausea and improve appetite?

a. Dronabinol.
b. Haloperidol.
c. Compazine.
d. Metoclopramide.

11. Following a stroke, a patient had progressed well but has become increasingly unwilling to carry out exercises or participate in activities of daily living. The patient has not joined in any activities in the unit and increasingly stays in her room with the blinds drawn. These observations are probably an indication of

a. small strokes.
b. dementia.
c. depression.
d. boredom.

12. If a patient with metastatic breast cancer has informed healthcare providers that she wants a DNR order and no heroic measures to prolong life but the patient's son and daughter insist that all life-prolonging measures be carried out, the best response is to

a. tell the son and daughter that the patient has a right to make this decision.
b. arrange a family meeting so that the patient and children can discuss this issue.
c. tell the son and daughter that they have no legal standing since the patient is alert.
d. urge the patient to tell her children not to interfere.

13. If using the ask-tell-ask framework to educate a patient about self-care, the advanced practice registered nurse would begin by

a. waiting for the patient to ask a question.
b. providing information and asking the patient to repeat it back.
c. asking the patient to write down a number of questions.
d. asking the patient what he/she knows and wants to know.

14. The advanced practice registered nurse has completed a history and exam of a palliative care patient and produced a problem list of nursing diagnoses that includes:

- Latex allergy response.
- Deficient fluid volume.
- Spiritual distress.
- Defensive coping.
- Anxiety.

When applying Maslow's Hierarchy of Needs, which order of priority (first to last) should be assigned to each problem?

a. (1) Deficient fluid volume, (2) latex allergy response, (3) anxiety, (4) defensive coping, (5) spiritual distress.
b. (1) Anxiety, (2) deficient fluid volume, (3) latex allergy response, (4) spiritual distress, (5) defensive coping.
c. (1) Latex allergy response, (2) deficient fluid volume, (3) spiritual distress, (4) defensive coping, (5) anxiety.
d. (1) Deficient fluid volume, (2), anxiety (3), latex allergy response, (4) defensive coping, (5) spiritual distress.

15. A hospice patient has increasing episodes of dyspnea, especially after exertion. The position of comfort that is most likely to reduce the dyspnea is

a. lying in bed with head of bed elevated to 45°.
b. sitting upright in chair with arms hanging loosely to the sides.
c. leaning slightly forward in a chair with arms supported.
d. leaning back in a recliner chair.

16. A patient with peripheral edema and venous ulcers may benefit from an Unna's boot. Which of the following is a contraindication for application of the Unna's boot?

a. Diabetes mellitus.
b. Peripheral arterial disease.
c. Ambulatory status.
d. Bedbound status.

17. The 5 key elements of the pain assessment include (1) words, (2) intensity, (3) location, (4) duration, and (5)

a. method/administration.
b. aggravating/alleviating factors.
c. frequency.
d. quality.

18. A 69-year-old patient with severe cognitive impairment has fallen and fractured her elbow. Which of the following pain assessment methods is most appropriate?

a. PAINAD.
b. FACES.
c. 1-10 scale.
d. LANSS.

19. The advanced practice registered nurse is conducting the timed-up-and-go test as part of gait assessment of a patient. The patient is able to stand from a chair with armrests, walk 3 meters, and turn and sit down. Which of the following times required to carry out these activities first indicates an increased risk for falls?

a. 7 seconds.
b. 10 seconds.
c. 14 seconds.
d. 16 seconds.

20. A male patient is being admitted for advanced cirrhosis of the liver and is hostile and angry, lashing out verbally at caregivers and refusing to cooperate. The best approach when conducting the history and physical exam is to

a. ask the patient to lower the voice and cooperate.
b. tell the patient that he cannot receive care unless he cooperates.
c. ask security personnel to stand by during the examination.
d. remain calm and patient, responding to the patient as appropriate.

21. The advanced practice registered nurse has begun to overly identify with the pain and suffering of patients and frequently finds that concerns about patients are interfering with personal life. The APRN often skips lunch and breaks in order to spend more time with patients and is beginning to have nightmares and trouble concentrating. The APRN is likely experiencing

a. depression.
b. compassion fatigue.
c. anxiety.
d. empathy.

22. If a patient with chronic bowel disease has developed persistent diarrhea, the treatment most indicated to control the diarrhea is

a. loperamide.
b. codeine.
c. diphenoxylate.
d. methylcellulose.

23. When utilizing the SPIRIT (Maugen) mnemonic (Spirit, Personal, Integration, Ritual, Implication, and Terminal events) as a spiritual assessment tool for a patient in hospice care, the first question to ask for the "S" or "spirit" part of the assessment is

a. "Does spirituality play a part in your personal life?"
b. "Are there any restriction in your religious convictions that affect your healthcare decisions?"
c. "How does your faith affect how you feel about death?"
d. "Do you have a formal religious affiliation?"

24. An obese patient with diabetes mellitus who underwent surgery for bowel obstruction 6 days previously and has had persistent abdominal distention and episodes of nausea and vomiting indicates a desire for palliative care. The patient complains of feeling a "popping" sensation at the incision site, and the advanced practice registered nurse notes a large amount of serosanguinous drainage on the dressing and separation at the center of the incision line with beginning intestinal evisceration. The initial response should be to

a. administer an opioid and keep patient comfortable with no further intervention.
b. place patient in semi-Fowler's position with knees elevated and notify surgeon.
c. explain to the patient what is happening and ask for guidance.
d. place the patient in supine position and cover the wound with dry sterile gauze.

25. A 76-year-old female patient who has generally been in good health has suffered a pathological fracture of the proximal femur. The patient states it occurred while walking, resulting in a fall. The most likely cause is

a. abuse.
b. multiple myeloma.
c. osteoporosis.
d. bone cyst.

26. When collaborating with a patient and family in developing the plan of care, it's important for the patient and family to understand

a. their rights and responsibilities.
b. their limitations.
c. the organization's philosophy.
d. the difference between goals and objectives.

27. A Native American patient has stage IV multiple myeloma and is under hospice care in an extended care facility. A staff nurse tells the advanced care registered nurse that, despite the diagnosis, the patient seems to have little pain. The patient does not complain or request pain medication although the patient has been lying in fetal position and refusing most food and drink. The advanced care registered nurse should advise the staff nurse that

a. the patient is probably comfortable without pain medication.
b. the patient may avoid outward expressions of pain.
c. the staff nurse should be more aware of patient needs.
d. the patient probably prefers to suffer rather than take pain medication.

28. A Middle Eastern hospice patient is being cared for in the home by the patient's sisters and daughters. During a home visit, the advanced care registered nurse notes that the patient has rows of circular slightly reddened areas up and down the back. The most appropriate response is to

a. notify adult protective services of physical abuse.
b. tell the family that hospice patients cannot receive cupping.
c. acknowledge the use of cupping on the patient.
d. provide supportive care for pressure sores.

29. A patient with progressive onset multiple sclerosis has chronic bladder dysfunction with bladder spasms, urgency, frequency, and stress incontinence. The patient takes extended release oxybutynin, which helps to reduce symptoms but not completely eliminate them. Which dietary/substance restrictions should the advanced practice registered nurse advise the patient to limit or avoid?

a. Simple carbohydrates (sugar, white bread).
b. Citrus fruits.
c. Apples and apple juice.
d. Caffeine and alcohol.

30. A family reports that the patient who raised Catholic has not attended Mass for 50 years. The patient is nearing death but remains responsive and has not requested a priest. The advanced care registered nurse should

a. assume the patient will not want to see a priest.
b. ask the priest on call to visit the patient.
c. ask the patient if he or she wants to see a priest.
d. ask the family if a priest should be called.

31. When educating a patient or family about disease and treatment, the first step is to begin by assessing the patient's

a. emotional status.
b. knowledge base.
c. experience.
d. physical condition.

32. Indications that the spouse of a patient who died is suffering from traumatic grief include prolonged period (≥60 days) of

a. expressing anger, bitterness, and blame regarding the death.
b. decrying negative habits of deceased (smoking, drinking).
c. focusing on occupational role.
d. talking frequently about the deceased.

33. A family member is concerned about the "death rattle" exhibited by a patient. When discussing administration of antimuscarinic agents, such as glycopyrrolate, what possible adverse effects should the advanced practice registered nurse consider?

a. Increased sedation, delirium, xerostomia.
b. Prolonged suffering, inability to communicate.
c. Insomnia, depression, anxiety.
d. Excessive sedation, respiratory depression, and itching.

34. When conducting a review of the literature as part of evidence-based research, the level of evidence that is based on a quasi-experimental study, such as a matched case-control study, would be categorized as

a. Level I.
b. Level II.
c. Level III.
d. Level IV.

35. A patient has osteomyelitis and an open draining wound in the proximal anterior thigh with copious amounts of purulent drainage. The wound has been requiring dressing changes 4-5 times a day. The most effective method of managing the wound care is to

a. apply alginate packing.
b. apply a pouch (such as Hollister® Wound Manager).
c. utilize negative pressure wound therapy.
d. applying absorptive dressings with cellulose fibers.

36. A female patient who has undergone surgery, radiotherapy, and chemotherapy for breast cancer has lost her hair but states she cannot afford to buy a wig. Which organization can the advanced care registered nurse refer the patient to for financial assistance for a hair replacement wig?

a. Songs of Love Foundation.
b. Association of Cancer Online Resources.
c. CancerCare.
d. American Cancer Society.

37. According to the American Geriatrics Society Guideline for the Prevention of Falls in Older Persons, if a patient has had one fall in the previous year

a. the patient should be assessed for gait and balance.
b. no further assessment is needed.
c. a full assessment, including vision, joint function, mental status, and neurological status, should be carried out.
d. the patient should be referred to a geriatric specialist.

38. If a patient receiving abdominal radiation has 7-9 loose stools daily with severe cramping and some incontinence, according to the National Cancer Institute Scale of Severity of Diarrhea, the patient's score would be

a. 1.
b. 2.
c. 3.
d. 4.

39. A palliative care patient with multiple sclerosis is increasingly immobile and spends most of the time in bed. Which of the following scores (range 6 to 23) on the Braden Scale is the breakpoint for risk of pressure ulcer?

a. ≤8.
b. ≤12.
c. ≤16.
d. ≤18.

40. A 68-year-old patient has appeared depressed, so the advance practice registered nurse assesses the patient with the Geriatric Depression Scale, which comprises 15 questions. How many "yes" answers are needed to indicate depression?

a. 4.
b. 6.
c. 8.
d. 12.

41. When conducting the history and physical exam of a military veteran who served in the Vietnam conflict, which of the following is a concern that applies primarily to only this population of veterans?

a. PTSD.
b. Shrapnel injuries.
c. Substance abuse.
d. Agent orange-associated illnesses.

42. If a dying patient tells the nurse that she has been seeing her mother, who has been deceased for many years, the most appropriate response is

a. "Does seeing your mother comfort or frighten you?"
b. "You are just dreaming."
c. "I'm sure your mother is watching over you."
d. "It's probably because of the medicine."

43. Which of the following unique needs may need to be addressed in the plan of care for homeless patients?

a. Fall and dysphagia precautions.
b. PTSD interventions.
c. Lice and malnutrition.
d. Drug-seeking behaviors.

44. A patient who completed a course of mantle radiation therapy for Hodgkin's disease 20 years previously has developed increasing weakness and shortness of breath on exertion. Because of the patient's previous radiation therapy, the patient is especially at risk of

a. pancreatic cancer.
b. breast and lung cancer.
c. liver cancer.
d. colon and rectal cancer.

45. The advance practice registered nurse has taken an active role in developing a support group for patients with Parkinson's disease to help them cope with their disease and delay progression. The group meets weekly at a local community center, and the APRN serves as the group facilitator. This type of preventive program is classified as

a. primary.
b. secondary.
c. tertiary.
d. quaternary.

46. A 17-year-old patient with AIDS and pneumonia is medically unstable and his parents have broached the subject of end-of-life decisions with him; however, the patient has steadfastly refused to discuss the issue, becoming quite agitated and stating that he is not going to "commit suicide." The parents are unsure how to respond. The APRN advises the parents to

a. remain supportive and wait for the patient's readiness to discuss end-of-life.
b. explain the difference between end-of-life decisions and suicide.
c. urge the patient to participate in some decision-making.
d. tell the patient that they will make the decisions for him.

47. A 15-year-old patient with leukemia tells the APRN that she wants to fill out a living will so that her parents will not have to make decisions about her end-of-life care by themselves. A document that is appropriate for adolescent patients is

a. *Five Wishes®.*
b. *Voicing My Choices®.*
c. *My Wishes®.*
d. *Willmaker Plus®.*

48. A 48-year-old patient with myasthenia gravis had been fairly stable but after a recent bout of gastroenteritis, the patient has experienced a marked weakening of muscles. The APRN notes tachypnea, a single-breath-count test result of 14, and oxygen saturation of 95%. This likely indicates

a. normal respiratory status for MG.
b. atelectasis.
c. pneumonia.
d. impeding respiratory failure.

49. A hospice patient who has been taking oral morphine to control the pain of pancreatic cancer reports little relief of constant pain, so the patient is to receive ketamine to relieve pain along with lorazepam once or twice daily in addition to the opioid. When ketamine is administered parenterally, the dosage of the opioid should

a. be reduced by 25-50%.
b. remain unchanged.
c. be increased by 25%.
d. be increased by 50%.

50. A hospice patient asks if the advance practice registered nurse or doctor can give her an overdose to cause her death because she is tired of suffering pain. The most appropriate initial response is:

a. "It's illegal for nurses and doctors to give overdoses to cause death."
b. "You don't really mean that!"
c. "Let's work together to better control your pain."
d. "You should talk to the doctor about that."

51. A 26-year-old male with no advance directive suffered a traumatic brain injury that left him in a vegetative state on life support. The patient's mother, sister, best friend, and fiancée are present. Which family member or other person can legally make the decision to withdraw life support?

a. Friend.
b. Sister.
c. Mother.
d. Fiancée.

52. The principle of the double effect refers to the idea that

a. drugs may not be used to control pain if they hasten death.
b. drugs may be used to control pain even if they hasten death.
c. drugs should not be administered in order to hasten death.
d. drugs can be administered in order to hasten death.

53. A patient with amyotrophic lateral sclerosis is no longer able to breathe independently but has elected to be extubated, understanding that this will lead to death. In addition to an opioid to relieve dyspnea, which other medication is usually administered?

a. Benzodiazepine.
b. Antipsychotic.
c. SSRI.
d. Atypical antipsychotic.

54. A patient with end-stage liver disease has made the decision to voluntarily stop eating and drinking (VSED) to hasten death, and the patient's family is supportive of this decision. What action should the advance practice registered nurse take?

a. Notify adult protective services.
b. Provide supportive care.
c. Advise the patient that VSED is an act of suicide.
d. Discontinue services to the patient.

55. A 50-year-old patient receiving chemotherapy complains that her biggest problem is managing her home and family while dealing with fatigue. Which of the following referrals may most benefit the patient?

a. Nutritionist.
b. Physical therapist.
c. Psychologist.
d. Occupational therapist.

56. The advanced practice registered nurse notes that a team member usually prefers to work alone and makes excuses for not delegating more of his workload. The team member frequently takes overtime shifts when the unit is shorthanded, but is increasingly short-tempered and complains of fatigue and headaches. The team member is likely to experience

a. burnout.
b. advancement.
c. ostracism.
d. injury.

57. When educating an 80-year-old patient about self-care and pain control, the teaching strategy that is most useful is to

a. review study skills.
b. allow ample time for learning and practicing.
c. utilize role-playing.
d. utilize problem-centered learning.

58. An advanced practice registered nurse has accepted a position in a different hospital and is in the "being" stage of role transition after 6 months in the position. This stage is characterized by

a. emotional lability and recognition of limitations.
b. acceptance of the new role.
c. increase in knowledge and self-doubt.
d. limited problem-solving skills.

59. A patient with COPD is recovering from pneumonia and has spent much of the day in bed with the curtains drawn and appears to have been crying. The most appropriate response is:

a. "You seem upset."
b. "Why are you crying?"
c. "Please, tell me what is bothering you."
d. "I'm sure everything will be OK."

60. When the advanced practice registered nurse (sender) is talking (transmission) and giving information (message) to a patient (recipient), communication is most dependent on the

a. situation.
b. sender.
c. message.
d. recipient.

61. Which of the following is most likely to be a barrier to effective communication?

a. The advanced practice registered nurse is nervous and speaks in a high pitch.
b. The advanced practice registered nurse speaks in a cheerful voice.
c. The advanced practice registered nurse rubs the hands together when speaking.
d. The advanced practice registered nurse leans toward the patient when speaking.

62. The advanced practice registered nurse frequently listens attentively to others and gives honest opinions, often beginning with "I" statements, such as "I would like to consider a different approach," and asking for opinions of others: "How do you feel about that?" The type of communication that the APRN is exhibiting is

a. passive.
b. aggressive.
c. neutral.
d. assertive.

63. According to the Joint Commission's "do not use" list, which of the following orders is documented correctly?

a. Levothyroxine .112 mg PO q AM.
b. Hydrochlorothiazide 12.5 mg PO q AM.
c. Metoprolol 50.0 mg PO BID.
d. Fluoxetine hydrochloride 20 mg PO each AM.

64. What type of conflict is occurring when two healthcare providers disagree on the best method of carrying out a treatment?

a. Relationship conflict.
b. Task conflict.
c. Process conflict.
d. Intrapersonal.

65. When the advanced practice registered nurse is presenting evidence about research to a group of nurses, the advanced practice registered nurse should begin by explaining the

a. validity of the research.
b. reliability of the research.
c. type and purpose of the research.
d. applicability of the research.

66. If the advanced practice registered nurse has reported safety concerns (such lack of proper equipment to lift patients and lack of retractable needles) to the administration a number of times with no results, the agency with which the APRN can file a confidential report is

a. Food and Drug Administration.
b. Office of Compliance.
c. Occupational Safety and Health Administration.
d. Department of Health and Human Services.

67. If a patient who was depressed committed suicide while on the unit and this was not discovered for a number of hours, the appropriate method of determining where processes to safeguard patients failed is to

a. carry out a root cause analysis.
b. assign blame to the staff on duty.
c. survey staff regarding responsibility.
d. take no further action as the patient was depressed.

68. If an 8-year-old child has been hospitalized for a prolonged period because of burn injuries, which of the following promotes autonomy?

a. Encouraging the child to nap in the afternoon.
b. Providing video games to entertain the child.
c. Encouraging the parents to remain with the child.
d. Allowing the child to assist in removing dressings.

69. The advanced practice registered nurse notes that a long-time nurse frequently berates a new staff member in front of other staff about the person's lack of experience in providing palliative and hospice care. This is an example of

a. lateral violence.
b. vertical violence.
c. slander.
d. libel.

70. The trend in healthcare regarding adverse effects, such as central line-associated bloodstream infections (CLABSIs), is to maintain

a. equivalent rate with national average.
b. rate below national average.
c. rate below regional average.
d. zero tolerance.

71. The federal agency that regulates the protection of human subjects and requires informed consent for patients involved in research is

a. Occupational Safety and Health Administration.
b. Food and Drug Administration.
c. Medicare.
d. Administration for Children and Families.

72. A patient undergoing abdominal radiation is suffering from severe radiation-induced nausea. Which of the following drugs is most indicated?

a. Prochlorperazine.
b. Lorazepam.
c. Ondansetron.
d. Metoclopramide.

73. A 38-year-old patient with acute myelogenous leukemia began chemotherapy with the two-drug regimen of cytarabine by IV continuous infusion on days 1-7 and daunorubicin by IV push on days 1-3. Three days after initiation of therapy the patient exhibits a sudden increase in potassium level followed by hyperphosphatemia, hypocalcemia and hyperuricemia. The most likely cause for this reaction is

a. allergic response.
b. tumor lysis syndrome.
c. myelosuppression.
d. kidney failure.

74. A patient has hepatocellular carcinoma that is classified as Stage IIIB, T3, N1, MO. Based on this classification, the advanced practice registered nurse understands the extent of the cancer to be

a. solitary tumor ≤2 cm in dimension, no vascular invasion, no regional lymph node metastasis, and no distant metastasis.
b. solitary tumor <2 cm in dimension, vascular invasion, regional lymph node metastasis, and distant metastasis cannot be assessed.
c. solitary tumor >2 cm in dimension, vascular invasion, regional lymph node metastasis, and no distant metastasis.
d. multiple tumors or invasion of other organs, regional lymph node metastasis, and distant metastasis.

75. A 38-year-old, olive-skinned patient, who has a long history of frequently using tanning beds and has about a dozen scattered nevi, is diagnosed with melanoma skin cancer. A distant cousin also had melanoma. The most likely risk factor that resulted in the development of melanoma in this patient is

a. olive-skin.
b. genetic factors.
c. presence of nevi.
d. use of tanning bed.

76. A patient with metastatic pancreatic cancer is considering whether or not to take palliative chemotherapy in order to prolong his life and asks the advanced practice registered nurse about how long most cancers respond to the treatment before the cancer worsens. The APRN notes that the median duration of response usually varies from

a. 2-4 months.
b. 3-12 months.
c. 12-18 months.
d. 18-24 months.

77. Which of the following opioid drugs should be avoided for pain control in children?

a. Codeine.
b. Hydromorphone.
c. Morphine sulfate.
d. Fentanyl.

78. A patient with diabetes mellitus complains of severe burning and "electric shock" neuropathic pain in legs and feet. Which of the following treatments may be most indicated to relieve the discomfort?

a. NSAIDS.
b. Acetaminophen.
c. Opioids.
d. Anticonvulsants.

79. A patient has developed tolerance to morphine sulfate and is to undergo opioid conversion to a different drug. The first step in opioid conversion is to

a. use an equianalgesic table to determine the correct dose.
b. determine total dosage of analgesia in previous 24 hours.
c. increase the dosage of new drug over current dosage.
d. stop the current analgesia for 12 hours.

80. If a patient with inoperable lung cancer has persistent hemoptysis, which palliative treatment is likely to provide the most relief?

a. palliative sedation.
b. palliative chemotherapy.
c. palliative surgery.
d. palliative radiotherapy.

81. If a patient who has undergone radiation of the salivary glands is unable to eat a dry cracker without drinking water, this suggests

a. xerostomia.
b. dehydration.
c. radiation burns.
d. mouth pain.

82. A patient is receiving Reiki massage as adjunct therapy to promote relaxation and reduce stress and anxiety. Reiki massage is classified as a(n)

a. whole medical system.
b. mind-body therapy.
c. energy therapy.
d. bioelectromagnetic therapy.

83. Which of the complementary therapies has evidence-based studies showing it can help to relieve pain?

a. Homeopathy.
b. Acupuncture.
c. Music therapy.
d. Therapeutic touch.

84. For a patient receiving chemotherapy for cancer, which of the following most increases the risk of sepsis?

a. Thrombocytopenia.
b. Anemia.
c. Neutropenia.
d. Thrombocytosis.

85. A patient with Parkinson's disease is completing the Quality of Life Scale (QOLS) (Flannigan). QOLS score can range from 16 to 112. If the patient scores 70, this indicates

a. normal satisfaction with life.
b. below normal satisfaction with life.
c. above normal satisfaction with life.
d. suicidal ideation.

86. When delivering bad news about a patient's response to treatment for cancer, the first step should be to gather the patient and family, assure privacy, and then

a. ask if they prefer not to know bad news.
b. begin with a piece of good news to soften the blow.
c. provide an overview of the patient's condition and treatment.
d. assess the patient's/family's understanding of the condition.

87. When conducting the history and physical exam of a new patient, the patient has multiple complaints and keeps interrupting the advanced practice registered nurse to discuss more issues, some major (abdominal pain) but some very minor (hangnail). The best response for the APRN is to ask the patient

a. to just answer questions briefly.
b. to help prioritize problems.
c. to explain in detail each complaint.
d. to only report major problems.

88. When conducting a system-based physical examination, the usual order of examination begins with

a. skin, hair, and nails.
b. heart and neck vessels.
c. head face and neck.
d. eyes, ear, nose mouth, and throat.

89. When utilizing the DIAPERS mnemonic to assess causes of acute urinary incontinence in a hospitalized patient, the D refers to

a. dementia.
b. decreased sensation.
c. dehydration.
d. delirium.

90. A patient with multiple sclerosis is hospitalized with a severe exacerbation of the disease. The patient's vision is severely impaired and the patient has a pronounced increase in weakness and poor balance, preventing the patient from ambulating or attending to activities of daily living. The treatment of choice is usually

a. plasmapheresis.
b. watch and wait and symptoms usually subside spontaneously.
c. low dose corticosteroids (prednisone) for 3-5 weeks.
d. high dose IV corticosteroid (methylprednisolone) for 3-5 days.

91. A patient with chronic osteoarthritis in the left knee complains of mild to moderate pain and stiffness. The initial treatment regimen begins with

a. NSAIDS.
b. acetaminophen.
c. hyaluronidase injection.
d. opioid.

92. A 68-year-old patient complains of recent onset of severe muscle pain and cramping in the legs. The advanced practice registered nurse reviews the patient's medication list, which include acetaminophen, atorvastatin, probiotics, levothyroxine, and vitamin D-3. The APRN suspects that the cause of the muscle pain and cramping is the

a. acetaminophen.
b. levothyroxine.
c. vitamin D-3.
d. atorvastatin.

93. A patient with primary biliary cirrhosis complains of severe pruritus, and scratching has caused numerous lesions. The treatment that may provide some relief is

a. rifampin.
b. antihistamine.
c. UVB phototherapy.
d. emollients.

94. A patient is taking opioids for severe back pain related to bony metastasis and complains of constipation and scores 12 on the Constipation Assessment Scale (range 0-16). The patient has persistent nausea and vomiting that has limited fluid and dietary intake. The initial pharmacological intervention should likely be

a. bulk laxative, such as psyllium.
b. combination stimulant and stool softener, such as Peri-Colace®.
c. lubricant laxative, such as mineral oil.
d. bowel stimulants, such as bisacodyl (Dulcolax®).

95. A patient with pancreatic cancer is switching from oral opioids to transdermal fentanyl patches for round-the-clock pain control. Before applying the patch, skin preparation includes

a. cleansing skin with alcohol wipe.
b. washing skin with soap and water.
c. shaving hair at site.
d. clipping hair at site.

96. If imaging shows that a patient has an intestinal obstruction from a cancerous lesion at the duodenum, the signs and symptoms likely include

a. copious emesis of undigested food, succession splashing bowel sounds, but absence of abdominal pain or distention.
b. moderate emesis, hyperactive bowel sounds, and upper abdominal pain.
c. moderate abdominal distention, colicky cramping, and hyperactive bowel sounds.
d. marked abdominal distention, some emesis (late), borborygmi, and colicky pain in central and lower abdomen.

97. A patient with malignant ascites has had a PleurX® catheter inserted into the abdomen in order to drain ascitic fluid. The advanced practice registered nurse is preparing the patient for discharge and teaching the patient to carry out fluid drainage. The APRN should advise the patient to drain at one time a maximum of

a. 500 mL.
b. 1000 mL.
c. 2000 mL.
d. 4000 mL.

98. A hospice patient who had been incontinent of urine and vomiting frequently has become dehydrated as the patient's condition deteriorates. The patient's daughter is concerned that her mother needs IV fluids to keep her comfortable. What is the best response?

a. "IV fluids don't make patients more comfortable."
b. "IV fluids may cause pain and discomfort."
c. "IV fluids may just prolong your mother's suffering."
d. "IV fluids may result in more incontinence and vomiting."

99. A 56-year-old female patient has developed lymphedema of the left arm after total mastectomy, radiotherapy, and chemotherapy. When discussing risk reduction, the advanced practice registered nurse should stress

a. avoiding weight loss.
b. restricting exercise of arm.
c. infection control.
d. keeping arm elevated.

100. Which of the following support surfaces used to prevent pressure ulcers has low moisture retention and reduced heat accumulation as well as reduction in shear and pressure?

a. Powered low air loss surface.
b. Powered alternating pressure air surface.
c. Non-powered foam surface.
d. Non-powered air surface.

101. Scheduled toileting to control incontinence in palliative care patients should include

a. asking the patient to delay voiding to scheduled time.
b. suggesting the patient ignore the urge to urinate as long as possible.
c. restricting fluids throughout the day to 1000 mL.
d. asking the patient to attempt to urinate at scheduled intervals.

102. When describing a pressure ulcer and undermining, the location of the undermining is described according to

a. quadrant.
b. clock-face reference.
c. degrees of a circle.
d. position--top, bottom, right side, left side.

103. Which of the following dressing types is most appropriate for a necrotic full-thickness wound with a small amount of exudate?

a. Dry sterile gauze.
b. Hydrocolloid.
c. Alginate.
d. Hydrogel.

104. A caregiver reports that a patient with Alzheimer's tends to get up during the night and has gone out into the street on two occasions and wandered about the neighborhood before being found. The advanced care registered nurse should advise the caregiver to place

a. the patient in a memory care facility.
b. restraints on the patient.
c. latches at the top or bottom of doors.
d. alarms on the doors.

105. The advanced practice registered nurse speaks to a state medical commission reviewing nursing practice and outlines the preparation that advanced practice nurses have and their ability to function effectively without physician supervision, urging that advanced practice nurses in the state be allowed more autonomy. In regards to the profession of advanced practice nursing, the APRN is serving primarily in the role of

a. consultant.
b. advocate.
c. advisor.
d. educator.

106. A 56-year-old patient has demonstrated marked changes in personality and behavior and has increasing difficulty using and understanding language. The type of non-Alzheimer dementia that this likely represents is

a. fronto-temporal dementia.
b. normal pressure hydrocephalus.
c. Creutzfeld-Jakob disease.
d. dementia with Lewy bodies.

107. A 40-year-old male who has been diagnosed with Huntington's disease exhibits hyperkinetic chorea and frequently grinds his teeth. While the patient had been demonstrating eccentric behavior, the patient now exhibits signs of obsessive-compulsive disorder and depression and has become increasing sexually aggressive although this behavior remains manageable. On examination, the patient exhibits chorea and tics. While still able to ambulate, the patient's balance is staggering and gait is uneven. Which medication regimen may be most indicated to control symptoms?

a. tetrabenazine, antidepressant, and mood stabilizer.
b. memantine, anti-androgen, and benzodiazepine.
c. levodopa, benzodiazepine, and botulinum toxin.
d. tetrabenazine, levodopa, and mood stabilizer.

108. A patient with advanced Parkinson's disease is no longer ambulatory and has increased tremors, muscular rigidity, and dysphagia as well as increased dementia with impaired cognitive ability, executive function, and memory. When instructing the caregiver about patient needs and risks, the risk of most concern is

a. falls.
b. aspiration.
c. pressure ulcer.
d. constipation.

109. A patient with a history of alcoholism weighs 70 kg (154 lb.) and, despite chronic heart disease, continues to drink. If the patient is admitted in a stupor with blood alcohol of 140 mg/dL, how long does the advanced practice registered nurse expect it will take to metabolize the alcohol?

a. 3 hours.
b. 5 hours.
c. 7 hours.
d. 9 hours.

110. A patient with liver disease and long-term alcohol use has been referred to a therapist for motivational enhancement therapy. The patient completes the stages of change (cycle) and remains abstinent for 3 months and then suffers a relapse. According to the MET approach, the response should be to

a. tell the patient to try a different method.
b. chastise the patient for relapsing.
c. advise the patient on what to do to stop drinking.
d. encourage the patient to begin the cycle again.

111. A patient who has undergone long-term treatment for schizophrenia with antipsychotic medications has begun exhibiting persistent lip smacking, tongue protrusion, and eye blinking and repeatedly grabs at her hair. The most likely reason for these signs and symptoms is

a. neuroleptic malignant syndrome.
b. tardive dyskinesia.
c. psychotic break.
d. hallucinations and delusions.

112. If a patient is diagnosed with class III heart failure, the advanced care registered nurse expects that the patient

a. experiences discomfort on any exertion and has limitations in most ADLs.
b. has symptoms even at rest and has limitations in all ADLs.
c. has symptoms with exertion but none at rest with some limitation on ADLs.
d. is essentially asymptomatic.

113. Which of the following is characteristic of peripheral arterial disease?

a. Brownish discoloration about ankles and anterior tibial area.
b. Irregular ulcers on medial or lateral malleolus.
c. Constant severe pain in legs.
d. Moderate to severe peripheral edema.

114. When assessing a patient for perfusion of lower extremities, which of the following venous refill times is consistent with venous occlusion?

a. >3 seconds.
b. >20 seconds.
c. >30 seconds.
d. >40 seconds.

115. Which of the following pharmacological interventions is typically indicated to maximize perfusion and prevent clot formation?

a. antiplatelet agent (aspirin, clopidogrel).
b. vasodilator (cilostazol).
c. antilipemic (simvastatin).
d. hemorheologic (pentoxifylline).

116. The advanced practice registered nurse is assessing cholesterol levels. Which of the following values is of most concern?

a. LDL cholesterol 98.
b. HDL 62.
c. Triglycerides 320.
d. Total cholesterol 198.

117. The advanced practice registered nurse's prescriptive authority is regulated by the states nurse practice act, which permits the APRN to prescribe controlled substances. In order to do so, the APRN must first apply to

a. Centers for Medicare and Medicaid Services (CMS).
b. State Board of Nursing.
c. Food and Drug Administration (FDA).
d. Drug Enforcement Agency (DEA).

118. The advanced practice registered nurse is using the ankle-brachial index to assess peripheral arterial disease in a patient. The patient's ankle systolic pressure is 75 and brachial systolic pressure is 165 for an ABI score of 0.45. This score indicates

a. normal reading, asymptomatic.
b. pain, even at rest, limb threatening.
c. critical limb threatening.
d. severe disease, ischemia.

119. If a patient is to following the Senokot S® protocol for cancer-associated constipation, on the first day the patient should take

a. 2 tablets at bedtime.
b. 2 tablets BID.
c. 3-4 tablets BID.
d. 2 tabs at bedtime with 8 ounces magnesium citrate.

120. When using the Plan-Do-Check-Act method to solve a problem, a number of possible interventions are considered and one implemented on a trial basis. If during the "check" step of gathering and analyzing data to determine if the trial intervention is effective, the analysis shows that the intervention is not successful, the next step is to

a. Return to "Do" and pick a different solution to try.
b. Continue with the intervention and reassess.
c. Continue to "Act" and determine changes needed for complete implementation.
d. Return to "Plan" and make a list of new possible solutions.

121. A patient hospitalized with renal disease develops pneumonia. In order to be categorized as "hospital-acquired pneumonia" (HAP), the pneumonia must not be present on admission and must occur

a. 12 hours or more after admission.
b. 24 hours or more after admission.
c. 48 hours or more after admission.
d. 72 hours or more after admission.

122. A patient with chronic hypertension is to begin the DASH (dietary approaches to stop hypertension diet). How many ounces of lean meat, poultry, or fish should the person eat daily?

a. ≤6.
b. ≤8
c. ≤10.
d. ≤12.

123. When considering quality control issues, the 3 basic types of failures in an organization are

a. medicine-based, safety-based, and time-based.
b. medicine-based, treatment-based, and safety-based.
c. skill-based, rule-based, and knowledge-based.
d. skill-based, treatment-based and knowledge-based.

124. A patient hospitalized for renal failure is frightened she may die and upset, and tells the advanced practice registered nurse that her biggest regret is having to give a child up for adoption when she was young. The APRN should

a. document this information.
b. share this information with the physician.
c. share this information with team members.
d. keep this information confidential.

125. When interviewing a patient, the advanced practice registered nurse notes that the patient is tapping his foot, moving his legs, and fidgeting with his clothes. The APRN recognizes that these actions may indicate

a. anger.
b. despair.
c. nervousness.
d. embarrassment.

126. The advanced practice registered nurse must visit a number of different patients, administering medications and treatments. How frequently should the APRN document?

a. every 1-2 hours.
b. every 2-4 hours.
c. every 4-6 hours.
d. after each administration/treatment.

127. Which patient characteristic puts a patient at increased risk and may interfere with recovery and/or compliance?

a. Resiliency.
b. Vulnerability.
c. Stability.
d. Complexity.

128. If a patient has Broca's aphasia and can understand but cannot produce language, what can the advanced practice registered nurse do to help the patient communicate?

a. Provide picture charts.
b. Provide letter boards.
c. Ask the patient to shake his head for "yes" or "no."
d. Ask the patient to draw pictures.

129. A patient who has had frequent hospitalizations for heart disease develops severe diarrhea associated with *Clostridioides difficile* infection. What type(s) of precautions are indicated?

a. Standard only.
b. Standard and contact.
c. Standard and airborne.
d. Standard, contact, and airborne.

130. When conducting a history under Medicare documentation guidelines, which elements must be covered for a problem-focused history?

a. Chief complaint and history of present illness (1-3 elements).
b. Chief complaint only.
c. Chief complaint, history of present illness, and review of symptoms.
d. Chief complaint, history of present illness, review of symptoms, and pertinent past, family/ and/or social history.

131. The advanced care registered nurse is carrying out a needs assessment to determine what needs in palliative and hospice care are unmet. The first step is to

a. select data collection methods.
b. develop tools, such as questionnaires.
c. identify the population to be assessed.
d. train data collectors.

132. When conducting the history and physical examination of a patient, the advanced practice registered nurse leans forward when the patient is talking and nods the head, occasionally making comments and asking questions for clarification. This is an example of

a. assertive communication.
b. passive communication
c. active listening.
d. passive listening.

133. A stroke patient's family has elected to place the patient, who is no longer able to make decisions, on hospice care. Which 2 criteria must be met?

a. Palliative Performance Scale (PPS) ≤40% and evidence of active pulmonary aspiration
b. PPS ≤50% and serum albumin <3.5 g/dL.
c. PPS ≤50% and ≥10% loss of weight in prior 6 months.
d. PPS ≤40% and ≥7.5% loss of weight in prior 6 months.

134. If a hospice patient who is no longer responsive has developed coolness in the extremities, progressing from distal to proximal, this usually means that death will occur within

a. 1-2 hours.
b. 2-3 hours.
c. 3-4 hours.
d. 4-5 hours.

135. The most common cause of hiccups in palliative and hospice care patients is

a. nausea.
b. respiratory distress.
c. gastric distention.
d. constipation.

136. A patient with systemic lupus erythematosus has had some serious complications in the past few years, but recently the patient's disease has been stable; however, the patient has begun to complain of a wide variety of complaints, including poor appetite, headache, backache, insomnia, nausea, sore knee, diarrhea, and constipation. The patient does not appear sad but is more hyperactive than usual for the patient. The advanced practice registered nurse should assess the patient for

a. infection.
b. substance abuse.
c. hypochondria.
d. depression.

137. Which of the following herbal preparations should the advanced practice registered nurse advise a patient to avoid when taking immunosuppressant drugs?

a. Melatonin.
b. St. John's wort.
c. Ginseng.
d. Curcumin.

138. When using music therapy along with relaxation exercises to reduce a patient's anxiety, the best type of music is

a. orchestral.
b. new-age.
c. patient's preference.
d. opera.

139. A COPD patient may need continuous oxygen to relieve dyspnea when the PaO_2 and oxygen saturation reach

a. PaO_2 ≤50 mmHg or oxygen saturation ≤85% at rest.
b. PaO_2 ≤55 mmHg or oxygen saturation ≤88% at rest.
c. PaO_2 ≤60 mmHg or oxygen saturation ≤90% at rest.
d. PaO_2 ≤65 mmHg or oxygen saturation ≤92% at rest.

140. A patient who did not seek medical care for years after developing a breast lesion has a large fungating lesion that has enveloped the left breast with copious amounts of foul-smelling drainage. Which of the following may help to relieve the odor?

a. Hydrogen peroxide.
b. Dakin's solution.
c. Metronidazole gel or solution.
d. Buttermilk.

141. Which of the following diagnoses puts a patient most at risk for the development of anorexia/cachexia syndrome?

a. COPD.
b. CHF.
c. HIV/AIDS.
d. Cancer.

142. If a hospice patient complains of frequent nausea and vomiting, the advanced practice registered nurse should begin treatment by

a. assessing the pattern of nausea and vomiting.
b. reviewing the patient's medication list.
c. ordering lab work such as CBC and differential and basic metabolic panel.
d. ordering abdominal imaging, such as CT or MRI.

143. If a patient is to following the Senokot S® protocol for cancer-associated constipation and has not had a bowel movement after the first day, on the second day the patient should take

a. 2 tablets at bedtime.
b. 2 tablets BID.
c. 3-4 tablets BID.
d. 2 tabs at bedtime with 8 ounces magnesium citrate.

144. A 72-year-old patient with chronic heart disease has blood pressure readings that have stabilized at about 150/94. This is categorized as

a. normal.
b. prehypertension.
c. stage 1 hypertension.
d. stage 2 hypertension.

145. If a male patient has urinary incontinence that is characterized by small leakages of urine, difficulty initiating flow (requiring the patient to strain to urinate), and post-urination dribbling of urine as well as frequency, these signs and symptoms are consistent with

a. stress incontinence.
b. overflow incontinence.
c. urge incontinence.
d. functional incontinence.

146. A palliative care patient recently suffered a stroke. The patient has regained strength although some residual weakness remains as well as expressive aphasia. Additionally, the patient has some short-term memory loss and exhibits slow cautious behavior. The patient needs repeated instructions to carry out tasks and has difficulty with math. Which part of the brain is likely affected by the stroke?

a. Left hemisphere.
b. Right hemisphere.
c. Brain stem.
d. Cerebellum.

147. An overweight male patient with hypertension and heart disease has been diagnosed as having obstructive sleep apnea by nocturnal polysomnography. Treatment includes use of the CPAP machine. The patient reports to the advanced practice registered nurse that she uses the CPAP machine about 5 nights a week while sleeping but doesn't use it when he takes a one-hour afternoon nap because he sleeps in his recliner with his head slightly elevated. The APRN should tell the patient that

a. the patient is using the CPAP machine correctly.
b. the patient should use the CPAP machine if the nap is longer than an hour.
c. the patient must increase CPAP use to every night.
d. the patient must use the CPAP machine every night and for all naps.

148. A patient with Alzheimer's disease becomes increasingly agitated in the evening and gets in and out of bed at night, wanders about the house, and empties the drawers in her room repeatedly. The patient is experiencing

a. hypersomnia.
b. insomnia.
c. sundowner's syndrome.
d. hyperactivity.

149. A palliative care patient under treatment for throat cancer is receiving total parenteral nutrition (TPN) because of severe dysphagia. The patient exhibits signs of azotemia with evidence of dehydration (dry mucous membranes, decreased skin turgor) as well as increased BUN and urine specific gravity. Management should include

a. decreasing amino acids.
b. increasing dextrose concentration.
c. increasing lipid intake.
d. decreasing lipid intake.

150. When instructing a patient with chronic constipation in bowel retraining, the advanced practice registered nurse advises the patient that the best time to schedule defecation is usually

a. upon arising, 20-30 minutes before breakfast.
b. 20-30 minutes after a meal.
c. any time that is convenient.
d. at bedtime.

151. Protein-calorie malnutrition (marasmus) is common in patients with chronic illness and is characterized by

a. sudden weight loss with loss of visceral protein but retention of skeletal muscle mass.
b. gradual weight loss with loss of visceral protein but retention of skeletal muscle mass.
c. sudden weight loss with loss of visceral protein and skeletal muscle mass.
d. gradual weight loss with intact visceral protein but loss of skeletal muscle mass.

152. If the average person requires about 0.8 g of protein per kilogram daily, how much protein should a person with a wound have each day in order to promote healing?

a. 0.8 g/kg.
b. 1.0 g/kg.
c. 1.25-2.0 g/kg.
d. 2.0-3.0 g/kg.

153. A patient is admitted to the unit with a 7 X 10 cm coccygeal pressure ulcer. On examination, the advanced care registered nurse notes that the exudate is green and a strong foul sweet-smelling odor is present. The most likely infective agent is

a. *Proteus.*
b. *Pseudomonas.*
c. *Staphylococcus aureus.*
d. *Escherichia coli.*

154. An older patient who suffered a fall from a hospital bed, resulting in a head injury and scalp laceration, has a Glasgow Coma Score of 10. This indicates

a. coma.
b. severe head injury.
c. moderate head injury.
d. mild head injury.

155. A patient with cirrhosis of the liver has portal hypertension with ascites. The patient is especially at risk for:

a. hemorrhage.
b. heart attack.
c. stroke.
d. kidney failure.

156. A patient has the following arterial blood gas values:

- pH: 7.26.
- $PaCO_2$: 57 mmHg.
- PaO_2: 53 mmHg
- HCO_3: 22 mEq/L.
- Oxygen saturation: 84%.

What do these ABG results indicate?

a. Respiratory acidosis.
b. Respiratory alkalosis.
c. Metabolic acidosis.
d. Metabolic alkalosis.

157. A 72-year-old female underwent a CABG because of severe chronic coronary artery disease and has been recovering well, but on the second post-operative day the patient has an acute sudden change in consciousness characterized by language disturbance, disorientation, confusion, and visual hallucinations. The signs and symptoms are fluctuating. The most likely cause is

a. stroke.
b. dehydration.
c. electrolyte imbalance.
d. delirium.

158. A patient with a history of severe combat injuries, including amputation of the left arm and chronic back pain from shrapnel, also suffers from chronic alcoholism and amphetamine use and has refused substance abuse rehabilitation services. The patient comes to the office with complaints of eye pain. On examination, the advanced practice registered nurse notes that the patient seems confused and is ataxic when ambulating. These signs and symptoms suggest

a. hallucinosis.
b. Wernicke's encephalopathy.
c. Wernicke-Korsakoff syndrome.
d. ethanol overdose.

159. The advanced practice registered nurse notes that patients never seem to have adequate pain relief when opioids are administered by another nurse, and this same nurse frequently offers to work double shifts and take on extra patients. The APRN should suspect that the nurse is

a. especially dedicated to seriously ill patients.
b. making errors when administering drugs.
c. diverting drugs for personal use.
d. purposefully withholding drugs from patients.

160. If the advanced practice registered nurse is working with and supervising the clinical practice of a graduate student preparing to enter the field for a semester of study and providing feedback that helps to determine the student's grade, the APRN is serving in the role of

a. preceptor.
b. coach.
c. mentor.
d. instructor.

161. Which of the following indicates the need for a patient/family conference?

a. The patient feels his family are only interested in their inheritance.
b. The family members have unrealistic expectations of the patient.
c. The patient has opted to begin hospice care.
d. The family visits the patient daily and is actively involved in her care.

162. A patient has advanced pancreatic cancer that has metastasized to the bowel and liver. When the patient asks if having chemotherapy will prolong her life indefinitely, the healthcare providers agrees that this is possible even though the healthcare provider knows that chemotherapy usually only prolongs life a few months. The ethical principle that the healthcare provider has violated is

a. confidentiality.
b. nonmaleficence.
c. veracity.
d. beneficence.

163. If a patient is dying, in addition to analgesics, which of the following medications are usually administered as long as possible?

a. Antihypertensives.
b. Diuretics.
c. Hormones.
d. Antiemetics.

164. If a patient's family member administers an intentional overdose of a prescription opioid without the physician's knowledge (although the physician ordered the drug) in order to bring about a patient's death because the patient asks the family member to do so, this would be classified as

a. euthanasia.
b. homicide.
c. suicide.
d. physician-assisted suicide.

165. At what stage of clinical competence (Benner) should the advanced practice registered nurse first consider forming a professional development plan?

a. Novice.
b. Advanced beginner.
c. Competent.
d. Proficient.

166. The advanced care registered nurse is serving as a consultant to a home health agency regarding palliative care. When asked to carry out a consultation for a patient, the APRN's first step should be to

a. determine if the visit will be billable.
b. ask for the referring healthcare provider's assessment of the patient.
c. arrange for an appointment to visit the patient.
d. assess the appropriateness of the request.

167. A patient with persistent urinary frequency associated with overactive bladder has been treated with oral oxybutynin and tolterodine but both oral medications in regular and extended release forms resulted in severe dry mouth. The advanced practice registered nurse should recommend

a. increasing fluids.
b. discontinuing medications.
c. decreasing dosage.
d. switching to transdermal patches.

168. As a team leader, the advanced practice registered nurse presents a problem to the team and asks members to arrive at a solution although the APRN usually makes the final decision. This type of leadership is classified as

a. consultative.
b. democratic.
c. bureaucratic.
d. autocratic.

169. A 28-year-old patient with cancer is not able to work and her husband makes minimum wage. The patient has no insurance and requires expensive treatment. Which of the following resources is most appropriate for the patient?

a. Medicaid.
b. Free clinic.
c. Medicare.
d. Go-Fund-Me campaign.

170. An 80-year-old patient has developed constant dribbling of urine. The patient is no longer ambulatory and spends most of his time in bed or in a chair. Which of the following options is likely most appropriate?

a. Indwelling Foley catheter (urethral).
b. Indwelling Foley catheter (suprapubic).
c. Adult containment briefs ("adult diapers").
d. External condom catheter.

171. A patient has a stage III pressure ulcer. Which of the following is a contraindication for negative pressure wound therapy (NPWT)?

a. Draining wound.
b. Post debridement.
c. Exposed vessels.
d. Slow-healing wound.

172. A patient is at risk for venous ulcers because of peripheral venous insufficiency. Which class of compression stocking is most appropriate?

a. Class I.
b. Class II.
c. Class III.
d. Class IV.

173. After application of eutectic mixture of local anesthetic (EMLA) cream to the skin prior to placement of an intravenous catheter, the area should be

a. covered with plastic wrap.
b. left open to air dry.
c. covered with an absorbent dressing.
d. irrigated after 5 minutes to remove residue.

174. If a patient's treatment has not been covered by Medicare and the patient wants to file an appeal, the first level of appeals is a

a. hearing.
b. redetermination.
c. review.
d. judicial review.

175. An adolescent patient hospitalized for leukemia has been unfailingly cheerful and avoids talking about the disease. The patient is making plans for an upcoming dance at school even though the patient is severely immunocompromised. The defense mechanism that the patient is likely using to help cope is

a. repression.
b. sublimation.
c. denial.
d. suppression.

Answer Key and Explanations

1. A: While various drugs have been used to treat restless legs syndrome, drugs that are FDA-approved for RLS and that are usually well-tolerated are pramipexole (Mirapex®) and Ropinirole (Requip®). The initial dose of pramipexole is usually 0.25 mg PO 2-3 hours before bedtime with dosage increased in 4-7 days if needed. Levo-dopa sometimes causes worsening of symptoms over time. Cabergoline is associated with severe adverse effects, and gabapentin may provide some relief of mild to moderate RLS but is associated with numerous adverse effects as well.

2. C: Stage III. Skin damage from radiation is common but usually begins to heal after radiation is completed and usually completes healing within 3 months.

Stage I	Slight edema, inflammation, erythema, itching, burning, or pain.
Stage II	Dry, itching, and scaly skin, and epidermis beginning to slough.
Stage III	Moist, blistering skin, epidermis sloughed off, serous drainage, and increased pain (exposed nerves).
Stage IV	Permanent hair loss, atrophy, pigment changes, and ulcerations.

3. C: If a COPD patient on corticosteroids has friable skin and has developed a skin tear with complete loss of tissue, this would be categorized according to the International Skin Tear Advisory Panel (ISTAP) Skin Tear Classification as type 3:

- Type 1: Linear tear with skin flap that can be positioned to cover the open area.
- Type 2: Tear with partial loss of flap leaving some tissue exposed.
- Type 3: Tear with complete loss of flap leaving the entire wound surface exposed.

Preventive methods include wearing long sleeves to protect the arms and applying emollients to skin.

4. D: The factor that most indicates a risk of drug abuse or misuse after beginning chronic opioid therapy is personal/family history of substance abuse. Patients with this history should be educated thoroughly about risks and monitored carefully. Other risk factors for abuse or misuse include a younger age and psychiatric comorbidity.

5. B: A patient may be eligible for hospice care on diagnosis of small cell lung cancer if the patient chooses to forego treatment because the prognosis is so poor and the average life expectancy is about 2-3 months. Other diagnoses that also may make a patient foregoing treatment eligible include pancreatic cancer, which results in a life expectancy of 4-8 months, and brain tumor (such as glioblastoma multiforme) with a life expectancy of about 6-8 months.

6. A: If an 80-year-old non-diabetic patient with renal failure who has refused hemodialysis and is not a candidate for kidney transplantation has requested hospice services, the laboratory findings that support admission to hospice are creatinine clearance < 10 mL/min and serum creatinine >8.0 mg/dL. Requirements for diabetic patients with renal failure are slightly different: creatinine clearance <15 mL/min and serum creatinine >6.0 mg/dL. The patient must also have documentation that outlines signs and symptoms consistent with chronic or acute renal failure.

7. C: If a patient with AIDS has a CD4+ count of 24, a viral load of 110,000, and a 35% drop in weight, the Karnofsky Performance Scale score needed to qualify the patient for hospice care is less than 50, which indicates that the patient is in need of assistance with activities of daily living and requires frequent medical care. The KPS classifies patients according to their functional ability, and a low score indicates a low chance of survival.

8. B: When the advanced practice registered nurse stays with a patient and holds the patient's hand when the physician delivers bad news about the patient's prognosis, the APRN is acting on the ethical principle of beneficence. Beneficence is acting to benefit another person, and this can include providing comfort in times of distress as well as ensuring that treatments should ultimately benefit the patient even though they may result in adverse effects.

9. D: If the advanced practice registered nurse is using the Palliative Performance Scale to assess a patient with severe heart disease and finds the patient is now completely bedridden, requires total care, oral intake of both food and fluids is reduced, and the patient is responsive but very drowsy, the PPS would be 30. Once a patient becomes bedridden, the highest possible score is 30. Scores of 50 and below indicate that disease is extensive and condition deteriorating.

10. A: If a 46-year-old male with HIV/AIDS has anorexia and marked weight loss, the drug that is indicated to relieve nausea and improve appetite is dronabinol. The usual initial dosage for adults is 2.5 mg PO before lunch and dinner or 2.5 mg PO in a single dose in the evening. The dosage may be gradually increased to 20 mg daily in divided doses if necessary. Dronabinol is a cannabinoid and is also used to relieve chemotherapy-associated nausea and vomiting.

11. C: If, following a stroke, a patient had progressed well but has become increasingly unwilling to carry out exercises or participate in activities of daily living, and the patient has not joined in any activities in the unit and increasingly stays in her room with the blinds drawn, these observations may likely be an indication of depression. Depression is common in those with chronic disease, especially if the disease involves disabilities that limit mobility.

12. B: If a patient with metastatic breast cancer has informed healthcare providers that she wants a DNR order and no heroic measures to prolong life but the patient's son and daughter insist that all life-prolonging measures be carried out, the best response is to arrange a family meeting so that the patient and children can discuss this issue. Both the patient and her children need to express their reasoning and their feelings about the patient's condition and treatment.

13. D: If using the ask-tell-ask framework to educate a patient about self-care, the advanced practice registered nurse would begin by asking the patient what the patient already knows about the condition and needs and what the patient wants to know. When the patient responds, the APRN tells the patient the information needed or wanted and then asks if the patient still has more questions or needs more information, continuing the cycle of ask-tell-ask.

14. A: If the advanced practice nurse has completed a history and exam of a palliative care patient and produced a problem list, when applying Maslow's Hierarchy of Needs, the order of priority is:

1	Physiological (Basic life-sustaining needs)	Deficient fluid volume
2	Safety and security (Physiological/Psychological threats)	Latex allergy response
3	Love/Belonging (Support, caring, intimacy)	Anxiety
4	Self-esteem (Sense of worth, respect, independence)	Defensive coping
5	Self-actualization	Spiritual distress

15. C: If a hospice patient has increasing episodes of dyspnea, especially after exertion, the position of comfort that is most likely to reduce the dyspnea is sitting in a chair and leaning slightly forward with the arms supported. The patient should be encouraged to take slow even breaths. Relaxation exercises may help the patient to breathe more slowly. A fan directed at the patient's face may help the patient to feel less anxious. Some patients may need oxygen for exertion if dyspnea is severe.

16. D: A contraindication to application of the Unna's boot, which is a compression therapy, is bedbound status because the purpose of the boot is to apply support to the muscles of the calf when the patient ambulates. Unna's boot may be used if the patient has peripheral arterial disease and/or diabetes. Impregnated gauze (commonly zinc oxide or glycerin) is wrapped around the foot and lower leg and allowed to dry and covered with a self-adherent wrapping.

17. B: The 5 key elements of pain assessment include:

- Words: Used to describe pain, such as burning, stabbing, deep, shooting, and sharp. Some may complain of pressure, squeezing, and discomfort rather than pain.
- Intensity: Use of 0-10 scale or other appropriate scale to quantify the degree of pain.
- Location: Where patient indicates pain is located.
- Duration: Constant or comes and goes, breakthrough pain.
- Aggravating/alleviating factors: Those things that increase the intensity of pain and those that relieve the pain.

18. A: If a 69-year-old patient with severe cognitive impairment has fallen and fractured her elbow, the pain assessment method that is most appropriate is PAINAD (Pain Assessment in Advanced Dementia). This scale assesses 5 elements: respirations (hyperventilation, tachypnea, Cheyne-Stokes), vocalization (silence, moan, groan, cry), facial expression (sad, frightened, grimacing), body language (tense, fidgeting, fist clinched, fetal position, combative), and consolability (inability to distract or console).

19. C: If the advanced practice registered nurse is conducting the timed-up-and-go test as part of gait assessment of a patient and the patient is able to stand from a chair with armrests, walk 3 meters, and turn and sit down, the time that indicates a risk for falls is equal to or greater than 14 seconds. The normal time needed to carry out the activities ranges from 7-10 seconds. Gait speed is also a consideration with gait speed of less than 0.6 m/second when walking 5 meters predicting limitations in mobility.

20. D: If a male patient is being admitted for advanced cirrhosis of the liver and is hostile and angry, lashing out verbally at caregivers and refusing to cooperate, the best approach when conducting the history and physical exam is to remain calm and patient, responding to the patient as appropriate. Cirrhosis is often associated with some degree of confusion, and the patient may be frightened and anxious, so speaking calmly and remaining empathetic and supportive is important.

21. B: If the advanced practice registered nurse has begun to overly identify with the pain and suffering of patients and frequently finds that concerns about patients are interfering with personal life, and the APRN often skips lunch and breaks in order to spend more time with patients and is beginning to have nightmares and trouble concentrating, the APRN is likely experiencing compassion fatigue. The APRN may need to take a break from work and participate in a stress management program.

22. A: If a patient with chronic bowel disease has developed persistent diarrhea, the treatment most indicated to control the diarrhea is loperamide, which is indicated for nonspecific diarrhea but should be avoided if the patient has grossly bloody stool or temperature above 38° C (101° F) or if infection with *C. difficile* or *Shigella* is suspected. Loperamide is usually given at 4 mg initially followed by 2 mg after each loose stool to a total of 16 mg per day.

23. D: The SPIRIT mnemonic (Maugen):

S	**Spiritual**	Formal religious affiliation?
P	**Personal**	Practices and beliefs? Spirituality in daily life?
I	**Integration**	Participation in a spiritual community and receive support?
R	**Ritual**	Specific practices and restrictions that affect healthcare choices?
I	**Implication**	Aspects of your spirituatlity you would like caregivers to keep in mind during care?
T	**Terminal events**	Faith affects decisions or feelings about death?

24. B: If a patient who has indicates a desire for palliative care complains of feeling a "popping" sensation at an abdominal incision site, and the advanced practice registered nurse notes a large amount of serosanguinous drainage on the dressing and separation at the center of the incision line with beginning intestinal evisceration, the initial response should be to place the patient in semi-Fowler's position, notify the surgeon, cover the wound with sterile saline soaked gauze, start an IV line, and administer oxygen. Palliative care does not preclude responding to emergent changes in condition.

25. C: If a 76-year-old female patient who has generally been in good health has suffered a pathological fracture of the proximal femur while walking, resulting in a fall, the most likely cause is osteoporosis. All women age 65 and older should be routinely screened for osteoporosis. Bone loss often exceeds 35% before the patient experiences symptoms. The DEXA scan is the imaging method of choice with results expressed as T scores. A T score of minus 2 (-2) is diagnostic of osteoporosis and indicates bone mass is 20% less than normal.

26. A: When collaborating with a patient and family in developing the plan of care, it's important for the patient and family to understand their rights and responsibilities. The advanced practice registered nurse should ask them what their goals and expectation are and what is most important to them. The APRN may ask the patient and family members to separately list those things that are important to them and then compare and discuss the lists because they may not always be in agreement.

27. B: If a Native American patient has stage IV multiple myeloma and is under hospice care in an extended care facility and a staff nurse tells the advanced care registered nurse that, despite the diagnosis, the patient seems to have little pain; and the patient does not complain or request pain medication although the patient has been lying in fetal position and refusing most food and drink, the advanced care registered nurse should advise the staff nurse that Native Americans often avoid an outward expression of pain. However, the patient's body language indicates discomfort.

28. C: If a Middle Eastern hospice patient is being care for in the home by the patient's sisters and daughters and during a home visit the advanced care registered nurse notes that the patient has rows of circular slightly reddened areas up and down the back, the most appropriate response is to acknowledge the use of cupping on the patient. Cupping is an ancient form of healing believed to rid the body of toxins and poses little danger to the patient if done correctly.

29. D: If a patient with multiple sclerosis has chronic bladder dysfunction with bladder spasms, urgency, frequency, and stress incontinence and takes extended release oxybutynin, which helps to reduce symptoms but not completely eliminate them, the patient should be advised to avoid caffeine and alcohol because they are bladder irritants and also promote diuresis. The patient should drink adequate water during the day but limit intake in the evening in order to decrease nocturia.

30. C: If a patient was raised Catholic but has not attended Mass for 50 years and is nearing death but remains responsive, the advanced care registered nurse should ask the patient directly if the patient wants to see a priest. Even lapsed Catholics who have not been active in the church may obtain spiritual comfort from the sacraments commonly referred to as last rites. The advanced care registered nurse should never make assumptions about a patient's spirituality.

31. B: When educating a patient or family about disease and treatment, the first step is to begin by assessing the patient's knowledge base and health literacy. Informed patients may already have a good understanding and may understand basic medical terminology while others may have little or no knowledge of health matters and may require much more intensive education geared toward their levels of literacy. The initial question may be, "Can you tell me what you know about your illness?"

32. A: Indications that the spouse of a patient who died is suffering from traumatic grief include prolonged period (at least 60 days) of expressing anger, bitterness and blame regarding the death. Other indications include avoiding talking about the deceased, avoiding social and occupational roles, showing signs of depressing, assuming some of the negative behaviors of the deceased (such as smoking and drinking), feeling and acting numb and dazed, and showing signs of impaired functioning (cluttered home, careless dress, poor hygiene).

33. A: If a family member is concerned about the "death rattle" exhibited by a patient, when discussing administration of antimuscarinic agents, such as glycopyrrolate (which can help to reduce the death rattle by drying up secretions), the possible adverse effects the advanced practice registered nurse should consider include xerostomia, increased sedation, and increased delirium. The nurse must balance these concerns against the stress the rattle may cause family members.

34. C: When conducting a review of the literature as part of evidence-based research, the level of evidence based on a quasi-experimental study, such as a matched case-control study, would be categorized as level III:

- Level I: Meta-analysis, randomized controlled studies.
- Level II: One or more well-designed study, may or not be randomized.
- Level III: As above.
- Level IV: Comparative non-experimental studies.
- Level V: Case reports and clinical examples but without empirical evidence.

35. B: If a patient has osteomyelitis and an opening draining wound in the proximal anterior thigh with copious amounts of purulent drainage requiring dressing changes 4-5 times daily, the most effective method of managing the wound care is to apply a pouch, such as the Hollister® Wound Manager. A skin barrier is applied around the wound, and the bag is attached, which has a drain that can be opened. The pouch is usually changed about every 4-7 days.

36. D: If a female patient who has undergone surgery, radiotherapy, and chemotherapy for breast cancer has lost her hair but states she cannot afford to buy a wig, the organization that the advanced care registered nurse can refer the patient to for financial assistance for a hair replacement is the American Cancer Society. ACS also provides financial assistance for durable medical equipment and transportation costs. The "Look Good, Feel Better" program provides assistance with techniques to minimize physical changes caused by treatment.

37. A: According to the American Geriatrics Society Guideline for the Prevention of Falls in Older Persons, if a patient has had one fall in the previous year, the patient should be assessed for gait and balance, including the get-up-and-go test. If the patient is steady, no further assessment is needed. If the patient demonstrates unsteadiness, further assessment to determine the cause is necessary. With multiple falls, a full assessment including history, vision, joint function, mental status, muscle strength, reflexes, neurological status, and cardiovascular status, should be carried out.

38. C: If a patient receiving abdominal radiation has 7-9 loose stools daily with severe cramping and some incontinence, according to the National Cancer Institute Scale of Severity of Diarrhea, the patient's score would be 3. Scale:

Score	#of stools above normal	Description
0	Normal stools	--
1	2-3	No other symptoms
2	4-6	Nocturnal stools and/or abdominal cramping
3	7-9	Severe cramping and some incontinence
4	10 or more	Grossly bloody stools and/or need for parenteral support

39. C: If a palliative care patient with multiple sclerosis is increasingly immobile and spends most of the time in bed. The score on the Braden Scale that is the breakpoint for risk of pressure ulcer is equal to or less than 16. The Braden Scale scores 5 areas with 1 to 4 points: sensory perception, moisture, activity, mobility, and usual nutrition pattern. The 6th area, friction and shear, is scored with 1 to 3 points. A score of 23 indicates minimal risk and 6 indicates a strong likelihood of developing pressure ulcers.

40. B: If a 68-year-old patient has appeared depressed, so the advance practice registered nurse assesses the patient with the Geriatric Depression Scale, which comprises 15 questions, 6 "yes" answers indicate depression. The Geriatric Depression Scale is a self-assessment tool to identify older adults with depression. The test can be used with those with normal cognition and those with mild to moderate impairment. Patients answer "yes" or "no" to the questions.

41. D: Agent orange-associated illnesses primarily affect veterans who served in the Vietnam conflict between 1961 and 1971, when the defoliant was used against combatants, exposing both the Vietnamese and American soldiers to potent pesticides (including dioxin) that may cause ongoing health problems. Agent-orange has been found to have teratogenic effects and to cause a number of different types of cancer, including leukemia and Hodgkin's lymphoma. Other associated diseases include diabetes mellitus, type 2, ischemic heart disease, Parkinson's disease, and peripheral neuropathy.

42. A: If a dying patient tells the nurse that she has been seeing her mother, who has been deceased for many years, the most appropriate response is: "Does seeing your mother comfort or frighten you?" Patients who are dying often report visits from loved ones who are deceased or from spiritual figures, such as angels or devils. The advanced practice registered nurse should neither challenge or support these perceptions but should encourage the patient to discuss feelings about them if the patient is still able to verbalize.

43. C: While homeless patients may face many of the same needs as other patients, the homeless are most likely to suffer from lice and malnutrition because of lack of access to adequate nutritional food and to bathing facilities. Homeless often share sleeping areas with others, so lice spread easily from person to person. Many homeless suffer from mental illness (such as schizophrenia) and are substance abusers, so general health may be very poor.

44. B: If a patient who completed a course of mantle radiation therapy for Hodgkin's disease 20 years previously has developed increasing weakness and shortness of breath on exertion, because of the patient's previous radiation therapy, the patient is especially at risk of breast and lung cancer. Patients treated for Hodgkin's disease have a 17% risk of developing another malignancy, including an increased risk of leukemia, with onset often within 4 years.

45. C: Support groups, such as one for patients with Parkinson's disease, are classified as tertiary prevention programs:

- Primary: Aims to prevent disease occurrence and may include educational campaigns (no smoking, seatbelts), vaccinations.
- Secondary: Aims to identify and reduce impact (screening mammograms, BP checks).
- Tertiary: Aims to prevent/delay disease progression (support programs). This is of primary importance in maintenance with palliative care/hospice patients.

46. A: Adolescents may be confused and indecisive about matters relating to end-of-life care; and some may, in fact, view end-of-life decisions as planning for suicide. The adolescent patient has been given an opening to discuss end-of-life care but has refused to do so and should not be forced to make decisions before the patient is emotionally ready. Decision-making can be especially difficult if a patient's condition is unstable because the patient may be experiencing a real fear that death is imminent. The parents should remain supportive and wait for the patient's readiness to discuss end-of-life.

47. B: If a 15-year-old patient with leukemia want to fill out a living will, a document that is appropriate for adolescent patients is *Voicing My Choices*®. The booklet allows the patient to indicate how the patient would like to be comforted and supported and who is to make medical decisions as well as the type of life support the patient wants. Additionally, there are sections where the patient can write personal notes, such as how the patient wants to be remembered and who is to have the patient's personal belongings.

48. D: If a 48-year-old patient with myasthenia gravis had been fairly stable but, after a recent bout of gastroenteritis, the patient has experienced a marked weakening of muscles, and the advanced practice registered nurse notes tachypnea, a single breath count test result of 14 (normal 50), and oxygen saturation of 95%. This likely indicates impending respiratory failure. An illness, such as gastroenteritis, can trigger a myasthenia crisis, which can severely impair respiratory function. With MG, the oxygen saturation level may remain adequate until the situation is life threatening.

49. A: If a patient is to receive parenteral ketamine to relieve pain along with lorazepam 1 mg once or twice daily in addition to the opioid, the dosage of the opioid should be reduced by 25-50% when ketamine is initiated. Ketamine can be administered orally, sublingually, or parenterally. An initial test dose, such as 25 mg, is often given and then the dosage is titrated upward until relief of pain is achieved. If PO or SL, doses may be taken 3 or 4 times daily. Continuous infusions are often used for SC or IV dosing. A number of different protocols are in use.

50. C: If a hospice patient asks if the advance practice registered nurse or doctor can give her an overdose to cause her death because she is tired of suffering pain, the most appropriate initial response is: "Let's work together to better control your pain." Patients who express the desire to die to escape pain often just want to be free of pain rather than really wanting to die, so the patient's pain control should be reviewed and stepped up until pain relief is adequate.

51. C: If a 26-year-old male with no advance directive suffered a traumatic brain injury that left him in a vegetative state on life support, the family member who can legally make the decision to withdraw life support is the patient's mother. If the patient were married, the wife would be first in line, followed by adult children, parents, and then siblings. Unless the fiancée has power of attorney, the person is unrelated and, like the friend, has no legal authority to make decisions for the patient.

52. B: The principle of the double effect is the idea that drugs may be used to control pain even if they hasten death because the intent is not to cause death but rather to relieve suffering. The Supreme Court (1997) affirmed the principle of the double effect. Most all religions also support the double effect. Patients are usually nearing death when they require such high doses that they may shorten life. In practice, sometimes alleviating pain reduces anxiety and may actually prolong life.

53. A: If a patient with amyotrophic lateral sclerosis is no longer able to breathe independently but has elected to be extubated, understanding that this will lead to death, in addition to an opioid to relieve dyspnea, a benzodiazepine is usually administered to help to relieve anxiety. The patient may also be administered oxygen. The patient should be supine with the head of the bed elevated to about 30° and family in attendance if possible.

54. B: If a patient with severe heart disease has made the decision to voluntarily stop eating and drinking (VSED), the patient has every right to do so under the law, and in states where physician-assisted death is not legal, this may be the only legal option available to the patient. The advanced practice registered nurse should remain supportive of the patient's decision, and should advise the family on comfort measures. Providing morphine and/or mild sedative may help to relieve feelings of hunger and thirst.

55. D: If a 50-year-old patient receiving chemotherapy complains that her biggest problem is managing her home and family and dealing with fatigue, the referral that may most benefit the patient is an occupational therapist. The occupational therapist can assess the patient's needs and recommend strategies to conserve energy as well as help the patient to recognize the need to make some changes and to set realistic goals during treatment and recovery. The patient may need help in establishing priorities.

56. A: If a team member usually prefers to work alone, makes excuses for not delegating more of his workload, frequently takes overtimes shifts when the unit is shorthanded, is increasingly short-tempered, and complains of fatigue and headaches, the team member is likely to experience burnout as these are all common factors. Burnout occurs when nurses become overworked and overwhelmed by the stress of the job and is a reason that many nurses leave the profession.

57. B: The approach to educating patients and family members should be adjusted according to their age and experiences. Teaching strategies for older adults includes:

- Allowing ample time for learning and practicing.
- Spending time chatting to get to know the individual.
- Eliminating non-essential information.
- Allowing the individual to set the pace.
- Remaining patient and supportive.
- Determining the individual's preferred learning style.
- Preparing materials that are age-appropriate.
- Providing written materials in large fonts and at appropriate reading level.

58. C: The "being stage" of role transition is characterized by increase in knowledge and self-doubt:

Stages of role transition (12 months)	
Doing (3-4 months)	Transition shock with emotional lability and self-doubt. Problem-solving skills limited.
Being (4-5 months)	Transition crisis, knowledge increases along with self-doubt. continued stress but increased awareness of role, feel unprepared for clinical situations.
Knowing (3-4 months)	Acceptance of the new role and recovering from some of the problems and stresses of earlier stages, explore and critique their new roles, gaining confidence.

59. A: If a patient with COPD is recovering from pneumonia and has spent much of the day in bed with the curtains drawn and appears to have been crying, the most appropriate response is: "You seem upset." This empathetic response acknowledges what is evident and recognizes the patient's feelings without prying into the reason. This response gives the patient the option to discuss the situation or not. Patients have a right to the privacy of their thoughts and emotions and should not be pushed to discuss issues.

60. D: When the advanced practice registered nurse (sender) is talking (transmission) and giving information (message) to a patient (recipient), communication is most dependent on the recipient. The recipient must be motivated to receive the message and must have no barrier, such as hearing impairment or emotional upset, that interferes with the transmission. The ability of the recipient to comprehend a message depends on many complex factors, such as cognitive ability, knowledge base, emotional status, sensory impairment, and health status.

61. A: The tone of voice can be a barrier to effective communication. For example, if the advanced practice registered nurse is nervous, this can raise the pitch of the voice, conveying nervousness and making the patient uncomfortable. People are more likely to listen to a cheerful voice (depending on the situation). While rubbing the hands together is a self-comforting measure, unless it is very obvious, it should not interfere with communication. The APRN should also make eye contact and stand or sit at a comfortable distance for the patient.

62. D: If the advanced practice registered nurse frequently listens attentively to others and gives honest opinions, often beginning with "I" statements, such as "I would like to consider a different approach," and asking for opinions of others (7"How do you feel about that?"), the type of communication that the APRN is exhibiting is assertive. The APRN is expressing an honest opinion directly while showing respect for the other person and disagreeing in an unthreatening manner.

63. D: According to the Joint Commission's "do not use" list, the following order is documented correctly: Fluoxetine hydrochloride 20 mg PO each AM. Abbreviations and items to avoid include:

- U or u for "unit and IU for in "international unit."
- QD, Q.D, qd, q.d., QOD, Q.O.D, qod, q.o.d.
- Trailing zero (but use leading zero)
- MS, MSO4, and MGSO4 for "morphine sulfate" or "magnesium sulfate."

64. B: When two healthcare providers disagree on the best method of carrying out a conflict, this is an example of task conflict. This type of conflict can lead to heated discussions but can generally be resolved through evidence-based research. Relationship conflict involves two or more people and personal feelings and discord and can lead to polarization as people take sides. Process conflict involves disagreement about responsibility to accomplish a task. Intrapersonal conflict occurs within the individual when personal needs are not met.

65. C: When the advanced practice registered nurse is presenting evidence about research to a group of nurses, the advanced practice registered nurse should begin with an overview that describes the type and purpose of the research and how it might apply to the organization. Then, the APRN should discuss the validity (format, methods used, external/internal validity), reliability (outcomes, problems), and applicability to target population (possible benefits and feasibility issues, such as costs).

66. C: If the advanced practice registered nurse has reported safety concerns (such lack of proper equipment to lift patients and lack of retractable needles) to the administration a number of times with no results, the agency with which the APRN can file a confidential report is the Occupational Safety and Health Administration (OSHA). OSHA and most governmental agencies provide a confidential method (fax, telephone, mail) to report lack of compliance with standards in order to prevent reprisals against the reporting individual.

67. A: If a patient who was depressed committed suicide while on the unit and this was not discovered for a number of hours, the most appropriate method of determining where processes to safeguard patients failed is to carry out a root cause analysis. In many cases, an adverse event is the result of a series of errors or system problems rather than one clearly identifiable process failure. The purpose or root cause analysis should not be to assign blame but rather to correct processes and prevent further sentinel events. Reviewers should remain unbiased and consider that system errors rather than human errors may be at fault.

68. D: If an 8-year-old child has been hospitalized for a prolonged period because of burn injuries, allowing the child to assist in removing dressings and participate in other care promotes autonomy. Children who are hospitalized may feel that they have no control over anything, so even small things, such as allowing the child to choose menu items, choose the site of a blood draw, or decide the time of dressing changes, are important for the child's sense of well-being.

69. A: If the advanced practice registered nurse notes that a long-time nurse frequently berates a new staff member in front of other staff about the staff member's lack of experience in providing palliative and hospice care, this is an example of lateral violence (AKA horizontal violence). Lateral violence is a form of bullying behavior that may occur among colleagues and may involve physical or verbal acts of abuse. Lateral violence can result in the victim losing self-esteem and motivation.

70. D: The trend in healthcare regarding adverse effects, such as central line-associated bloodstream infections (CLABSIs), is to maintain zero tolerance. The goal is no infections at all. This requires continued emphasis on preventive measures, proper procedures, and best practices, as well as ongoing training for staff members. The staff should have a clear understanding of actions that will be taken if zero tolerance policies are breached, such as through improper handling of equipment or failure to utilize correct hand hygiene.

71. B: The federal agency that regulates the protection of human subjects and requires informed consent for patients involved in research is the Food and Drug Administration (Code of Federal Regulations, Title 21, volume 1). Patients must be made aware of any risk of benefits, and compensation (if provided) must be outlines. Patients must understand that they can opt out of participation at any time without penalty because participation in research is always voluntary.

72. C: If a patient undergoing abdominal radiation is suffering from severe radiation-induced nausea, ondansetron is most indicated. Ondansetron is a selective serotonin (5-HT3) receptor antagonist (0.15-0.18 mg/kg orally or IV every 12 hours may provide some relief. Ondansetron is also used to prevent nausea and vomiting associated with emetogenic chemotherapy, with the medication usually administered 30 minutes before chemotherapy.

73. B: If a 38-year old patient with acute myelogenous leukemia began chemotherapy with the two-drug regimen of cytarabine by IV continuous infusion on days 1-7 and daunorubicin by IV push on days 1-3 and, 3 days after initiation of therapy, the patient exhibits a sudden increase in potassium level followed by hyperphosphatemia, hypocalcemia and hyperuricemia, the most likely cause for this reaction is tumor lysis syndrome. This life-threatening condition occurs when large numbers of cancer cells are destroyed and their byproducts are released into the bloodstream.

74. C: If a patient has hepatocellular carcinomas that is classified as Stage IIIB, T3, Ni, MO, the APRN understands the extent of the cancer to be a solitary tumor >2 cm in dimension with vascular invasion, regional lymph node metastasis, and no distant metastasis. With TNM staging, T refers too primary tumor, N refers to regional lymph nodes, and M refers to distant metastasis. Letters and number follow the TNM classifications: X means cannot be assessed, 0 means not evident, and numbers 1-4 indicate increasing size, number, or extent.

75. D: If a 38-year-old olive-skinned patient who has a long history of frequently using tanning beds and has about a dozen scattered nevi is diagnosed with melanoma skin cancer, and a distant cousin also had melanoma, the most likely risk factor that resulted in the development of melanoma in this patient is use of tanning beds. Other risk factors include large numbers of nevis (>100), first-degree relative history, previous skin cancer, and immunocompromise. Fair-skinned patients are more at risk than darker-skinned.

76. B: Palliative chemotherapy is often used with metastatic cancer to shrink the lesions and to extend the patient's life; however, these side effects may be very debilitating, so the patient needs to be aware of the tradeoff in quality of life for quantity. The median duration of response (the time during which the cancer responds to treatment until the cancer begins to grown again) varies depending on the type of tumor but is usually between 3 and 12 months.

77. A: Codeine is an opioid drug that is generally not recommended for use in children. Meperidine is also not recommended for children for pain control but it may be used to treat shivering. Children may receive morphine sulfate, hydromorphone, fentanyl, hydrocodone, and methadone. Dosage is lower than adults and usually calculated according to kilograms of weight rather than age of child to prevent overdosage.

78. D: Neuropathic pain, such as severe burning and "electric shock" pain, responds poorly to typical analgesia, including NSAIDs, acetaminophen, and opioids. Adjuvant medications, such as anticonvulsants (clonazepam, gabapentin, carbamazepine) may provide more relief. Other medications used for neuropathic pain include calcitonin, calcium channel blockers, capsaicin topical preparation, local anesthetics, NMDA antagonists, and tricyclic antidepressants.

79. B: Steps to opioid conversion include:

- Determine the total dose of analgesia during the previous 24 hours.
- Calculate the equianalgesic dose according to an equianalgesia table.
- If pain has been controlled, decrease the new medication dosage by 25% to 50% initially.
- If pain has NOT been controlled, increased the dosage up to 100% to 125% overcurrent equianalgesic dose OR rotate opioids at the equianalgesic dose.
- Observe patient carefully and titrate dosage up or down during initial 24 hours.

- Evaluate effectiveness and adverse effects, titrate as needed.
- Reassess effectiveness of new drug every two to three days.

80. D: If a patient with metastatic lung cancer has persistent hemoptysis, palliative radiotherapy provides control of hemoptysis in up to 80% of patients. Radiation, however, does pose some risk of adverse effects that the patient must consider in relation to the quality of life. The radiation may increase fatigue and cause local skin irritation and burns as well as GI upset, anemia, and immunocompromise.

81. A: If a patient who has undergone radiation of the salivary glands is unable to eat a dry cracker without drinking water (cracker test), this suggests xerostomia, which results from a change in saliva or decrease production. Pilocarpine is a nonselective muscarinic that increases saliva production, but it may result in increased perspiration, nausea, flushing, and cramping. Saliva substitutes may provide partial relief. Good mouth care is essential to prevent further irritation and development of caries.

82. C: If a patient is receiving Reiki massage as adjunct therapy to promote relaxation and reduce stress and anxiety, this treatment is classified as an energy therapy. Energy therapies are intended to affect the aura (energy field) that some believe surrounds living things. Therapeutic touch is also an energy therapy. Mind-body therapy includes support groups, meditation, music, art, and dance therapy. Whole medical systems include homeopathic, naturopathic, acupuncture, and Chinese herbal medications. Bioelectromagnetic therapy uses manipulation of magnetic fields.

83. B: Evidence-based studies have shown that acupuncture can help to reduce pain, and acupuncture is likely the most effective adjunct therapy and is widely used. There is no evidence to suggest that therapeutic touch can relieve pain although it may have a placebo affect and may help to relax patients. A number of studies of homeopathy have shown that it is generally not effective to treat anything. Music therapy may help to distract the person from pain and may relax the patient and reduce anxiety associated with pain.

84. C: For a patient receiving chemotherapy for cancer, neutropenia most increases the risk of sepsis. Normal neutrophil range is 50-60% of white blood cells. Risk is especially severe if the absolute neutrophil count decrease to <500/μL. Neutrophils serve as part of the defense of bacterial infections and typically increase, but chemotherapy may cause a decrease in neutrophils, usually about one to two weeks after beginning therapy because of bone marrow suppression. Patients are often asymptomatic until an infection occurs although some may feel fatigued.

85. B: If a patient with Parkinson's disease is completing the Quality of Life Scale (QOLS) (Flannigan) (scores range from 16 to 112) and scores 70, this indicates below normal (which is about 90) satisfaction with life. The QOLS is a self-administered test that assesses the patient's perception of the quality of life. Sixteen elements are scored from 1-7 (dissatisfaction to satisfaction). Categories include material/physical well-being, interpersonal relationships, activities, personal development/fulfillment, recreation, and independence.

86. D: When delivering bad news about a patient's response to treatment for cancer, the first step should be to gather the patient and family (and a spiritual adviser if appropriate), assure privacy and a quiet space, and then assess the patient's/family's understanding of the condition. This should be followed by a brief overview of the condition and treatment to date and a warning that the news is not good ("I'm sorry that I have some bad news"), followed by a pause to allow the patient/family to digest this news and respond or question before providing more details.

87. B: If, when conducting the history and physical exam of a new patient, the patient has multiple complaints and keeps interrupting the advanced practice registered nurse to discuss more issues, some major (abdominal pain) but some very minor (hangnail), the best response for the APRN is to ask the patient to help prioritize problems. This may help the patient to focus on problems that are more severe, although problems that seem minor (such as fatigue) may be an indication of a serious health concern.

88. A: When conducting a system-based physical examination, the usual order of examination begins with skin, hair, and nails because these are elements that can easily be assessed with minimal touching and through simple observation. The examination then proceeds generally from the head down:

- Head, face, and neck
- Eyes, ears, nose, mouth, and throat
- Breasts and regional lymph nodes
- Thorax and lungs
- Heart and neck vessels
- Peripheral vascular/lymphatic system
- Abdomen
- Musculoskeletal system (may include functional assessment)
- Genitourinary system
- Anus, rectum, and prostate

89. D: DIAPERS mnemonic:

D	**Delirium**	Acute delirium and the related confusion may cause acute urinary incontinence.
I	**Infection**	Especially urinary tract infection
A	**Atrophic urethritis**	May cause irritation and stress incontinence
P	**Pharmacy**	Many drugs increase urinary retention and stress incontinence.
E	**Excessive urine production**	May be associated with disease, such as diabetes
R	**Restricted mobility**	Inability to access toilet facilities
S	**Stoll impaction**	May block flow of urine

90. D: If a patient with multiple sclerosis is hospitalized with a severe exacerbation of the disease, and the patient's vision is severely impaired and the patient has a pronounced increase in weakness and poor balance, preventing the patient from ambulating or attending to activities of daily living, the treatment of choice is usually high dose IV corticosteroid (methylprednisolone) for 3-5 days. This may be followed by a tapering dose of oral steroid. Plasmapheresis may be used if the patient does not respond to the corticosteroids. H.P Acthar Gel (purified ACTH) is another treatment option.

91. B: If a patient with chronic osteoarthritis in the left knee complains of mild to moderate pain and stiffness, the initial treatment regimen begins with acetaminophen, which should be limited to 4,000 mg per day because of the risk of liver damage from high doses. NSAIDs should be reserved for more severe pain because of the risks (such as GI hemorrhage) associated with long-term use. If pain persists or condition worsens, the patient may benefit from hyaluronic acid injection or corticosteroid injection into the joint.

92. D: If a 68-year-old patient complains of recent onset of severe muscle pain and cramping in the legs and the patient's medication list includes acetaminophen, atorvastatin, probiotics, levothyroxine, and vitamin D-3, the advanced practice registered nurse should suspect that the cause of the muscle pain and cramping is the atorvastatin. Patients who develop muscle pain and cramping may be able to tolerate a different statin drug. Rhabdomyolysis, damage to muscle tissue, as well as liver damage may occur as rare side effects in some patients.

93. A: If a patient with primary biliary cirrhosis complains of severe Pruritus and scratching has caused numerous lesions, the treatment that may provide some relief is rifampin, which is usually used to treat tuberculosis but is often effective in relieving Pruritus associated with liver disease. The patient should also apply soothing emollients to relieve dry skin. Other treatments that may be considered for intractable itching include dronabinol (a cannabinoid), UBV phototherapy, and opioid antagonists, such as naloxone.

94. B: Opioid-associated constipation often responds best to a combination stimulant and stool softener, such as Peri-Colace. Alternately, two separate medications (one a stool softener and one a stimulant) may be administered. Bulk laxatives should be avoided without adequate fluid intake. Mineral oil interferes with absorption of fat-soluble vitamins. Bowel stimulants, such as bisacodyl, are relatively harsh. The Constipation Assessment Scale (range 0-16) includes 8 questions about bowel status for which the patient scores from 0 (no problem), to 1 (some problem), to 2 (severe problem).

95. D: If a patient with pancreatic cancer is switching from oral opioids to transdermal fentanyl patches for round-the-clock pain control, before applying the patch, skin preparation includes clipping hair at the site (avoid shaving, which may irritate skin) and cleansing the skin with water only and allowing the skin to dry completely before application of the patch. No soap, oils, emollients, or alcohol should be used on the skin as these may cause skin irritation or interfere with adherence so that the patch falls off.

96. A: If imaging shows that a patient has an intestinal obstruction from a cancerous lesion at the duodenum, the signs and symptoms likely include copious emesis of undigested food (with no evidence of bile) after eating, succession splashing bowel sounds in the left upper quadrant but generally absence of abdominal pain or distention. If the condition persists untreated, the patient may show signs of dehydration and muscle wasting. The stomach may begin to dilate and excessive peristaltic action may be evident.

97. C: If a patient with malignant ascites has had a PleurX® catheter inserted into the abdomen in order to drain ascitic fluid and the advanced practice registered nurse is preparing the patient for discharge and teaching the patient to carry out fluid drainage, the APRN should advise the patient to drain at one time a maximum of 2000 mL. While paracentesis in the hospital may drain up to 5000 mL, the home patient will be draining more frequently and fluid should not build up to this extent. The patient should practice using aseptic technique to prevent infection and should understand the drainage schedule and signs of fluid buildup.

98. D: If a hospice patient who had been incontinent of urine and vomiting frequently has become dehydrated as the patient's condition deteriorates, but the patient's daughter is concerned that her mother needs IV fluids to keep her comfortable, the best response: "IV fluids may result in more incontinence and vomiting." While it's also true that IV fluids may cause pain and may prolong suffering and will probably not make the patient more comfortable, the incontinence and vomiting are concrete examples that the daughter has experienced and can likely more readily accept.

99. C: If a 56-year-old female patient has developed lymphedema of the left arm after total mastectomy, radiotherapy, and chemotherapy, when discussing risk reduction, the advanced practice registered nurse should stress infection control. Infection is the most common complication of lymphedema, so the patient needs to be aware of the need to examine the skin carefully for any cuts or abrasions, to avoid blood draws from that arm, and to avoid garments that may rub or irritate skin.

100. A: The support surfaces used to prevent pressure injuries that have low moisture retention and reduced heat accumulation as well as reduction in shear and pressure include the powered low air loss surface and the powered air fluidized surface. However, both of these surfaces are expensive. The low air loss surface is suitable for pressure reduction in the hospital and at home and fits on top of the existing mattress, but the powered air fluidized surface requires a special bed frame that is filled with silicone-coated glass beads through which air is pumped. Alternating pressure air surfaces primarily redistribute pressure via cyclic inflation and deflation; they do not manage heat or moisture unless they include a low–air–loss feature. Nonpowered foam and nonpowered air surfaces provide pressure redistribution but lack powered airflow for climate control, so they do not meet the requirements of low moisture retention and reduced heat accumulation.

101. D: Scheduled toileting to control incontinence in palliative care patients should include asking the patient to attempt to urinate at scheduled intervals, such as every 2-3 hours or after each meal and at bedtime. If possible, it's best to try to approximate the schedule to the patient's usual urination times. The patient should not be expected to restrict fluids throughout the day but may be asked to restrict fluids near bedtime if nocturia is a problem. The patient should not be asked to delay voiding or ignore the urge to urinate.

102. B: When describing a pressure ulcer and undermining, the location of the undermining is described according to clock-face reference. For example, a description may be stated as "Undermining of 2 cm width extending from 1 to 3 o'clock." If the undermining is open to the wound, it may be measured by inserting a sterile swab. If it is not open to the wound, the tissue may feel boggy when palpated. The wound itself should be measured in centimeters at its widest length and width: "6 X 8 cm."

103. D: Hydrogel dressings, such as AquaForm®, are most appropriate for a necrotic full-thickness wound with a small amount of exudate. These dressings, which may come in various forms (pates, sheets, strips), are applied directly to the wound and are then covered with a secondary dressing. Hydrogel dressings are effective to provide warmth and moisture to the wound and autolysis to aid in the removal of the necrotic tissue. Hydrogel dressings are not appropriate for wounds with large amounts of exudate.

104. C: If a caregiver reports that a patient with Alzheimer's tends to get up during the night and has gone out into the street on two occasions and wandered about the neighborhood before being found, the advanced care registered nurse should advise the caregiver to place latches at the top or bottom of doors as patients with Alzheimer's rarely look for the latches in those areas. Door alarms, especially those that are loud, are often very frightening for patients, and restraints should be avoided.

105. B: If the advanced practice registered nurse speaks to a state medical commission reviewing nursing practice and outlines the preparation that advanced practice nurses have and their ability to function effectively without physician supervision, urging that advanced practice nurses in the state be allowed more autonomy, the APRN is serving primarily in the role of advocate for advanced practice nursing. Advancing opportunities for advanced practice nurses is especially important in areas with a shortage of physicians as the APRN can fill a vital role in providing medical care.

106. A: If a 56-year-old patient has demonstrated marked changes in personality and behavior and has increasing difficulty using and understanding language, the type of non-Alzheimer dementia that this likely represents is fronto-temporal dementia. Onset of FTD is most common in people who are in their 50s. Patients may develop disinhibited and/or rigid ritualistic behaviors, and some may develop increased interest (sometimes inappropriate) in sex and may crave sweet and/or fatty foods.

107. A: For a patient with Huntington's disease whose symptoms include hyperkinetic chorea, obsessive-compulsive disorder, and depression, the medication regimen that is most indicated include tetrabenazine (FDA approved to treat chorea), antidepressant, and mood stabilizer. Memantine usually shows little results, and levodopa is used to treat hypokinetic rigidity (not chorea). Some patients act sexually inappropriate while others lose interest in sex, but anti-androgens are usually reserved for those who become so sexually aggressive that they place others at risk.

108. B: While falls, pressure ulcers, and constipation are all concerns for patients with advanced Parkinson's disease, the greatest concern is aspiration because the most common cause of death in Parkinson's disease is aspiration pneumonia associated with increasing dysphagia. Unfortunately, there is no satisfactory medical treatment. The patient may benefit from exercises to strengthen the muscles of swallowing and should eat soft foods in small amount and while sitting upright. Thickening liquids may help prevent aspiration.

109. C: If a patient with a history of alcoholism weighs 70 kg (154 lb.) and, despite chronic heart disease, continues to drink, and the patient is admitted in a stupor with blood alcohol of 140 mg/dL, it should take approximately 7 hours (20 mg/dL per hour) to metabolize the alcohol. For a patient weighing 70 kg, one drink (1 ounce liquor, 4-6 ounces of wine, or 12 ounces of beer) usually raises the blood alcohol level by about 25 mg/dL (35 mg/dL if the person weighs 50 kg).

110. D: If a patient with liver disease and long-term alcohol use has been referred to a therapist for motivational enhancement therapy, completes the stages of change (cycle), remains abstinent for 3 months, and then suffers a relapse, according to the MET approach, the response should be to encourage (not criticize, label, or advise) the patient to start the cycle again. Stages of change:

Pre-contemplation	No desire to change behavior.
Contemplation	Considers positive and negative aspects of drug/alcohol use.
Determination	Decides to change.
Action	Modifies behavior over time (2-6 months).
Maintenance	Remains abstinent.
Relapse	Begins cycle again. (Several relapses are common).

111. B: If a patient who has undergone long-term treatment for schizophrenia with antipsychotic medications has begun exhibiting persistent lip smacking, tongue protrusion, and eye blinking and repeatedly grabs at her hair, the most likely reason for these signs and symptoms is tardive dyskinesia. This chronic syndrome associated with use of antipsychotic drugs most affects older adults. Patients with schizophrenia are also especially at risk because of treatments and substance abuse. In about 50% of patients, even stopping the medication will not relieve the symptoms.

112. A: If a patient is diagnosed with class III heart failure, the advanced care registered nurse expects that the patient experiences discomfort of any exertion and has limitations in most ADLs.

Class I	Essentially asymptomatic during normal activities with no pulmonary congestion or peripheral hypotension. No restriction on activities, good prognosis.
Class II	Symptoms with some physical exertion, usually absent at rest, some limitations of ADLs. Slight pulmonary edema may be evident by basilar rales. Good prognosis.
Class III	Obvious limitations of ADLs and discomfort on any exertion, prognosis is fair.
Class IV	Symptoms at rest, poor prognosis.

113. C: Peripheral arterial disease is characterized by pain that may range from intermittent to severe constant pain. Pedal pulses are generally very weak or absent. The foot may be rubor on dependency and pale on elevation, and the skin may be pale, shiny, and cool with hair loss on foot and toes. Nails may be thick and ridged. If ulcers are present, they are often deep, painful, necrotic, and circular and typically occur in toe tips, toe webs, heels, and pressure areas. Edema is usually absent or minimal.

114. B: When assessing a patient for perfusion of lower extremities, the venous refill time that is consistent with venous occlusion is greater than 20 seconds. To assess venous refill time, the advanced practice registered nurse should direct the patient to lie in supine position for a few minutes and then quickly place the patient in sitting position with the feet dependent. The APRN observes the vessels in the dorsal surface of the foot and counts the seconds until the veins have normal filling.

115. A: The pharmacological intervention that is typically indicated to maximize perfusion and prevent clot formation is an antiplatelet agent, such as aspirin or clopidogrel (Plavix®). Current recommendations for aspirin preventive therapy include low dose (81 mg) aspirin daily for males ages 45-79 and female ages 55-79 if potential reduction in myocardial infarcts in females and ischemic strokes in males outweigh risks of gastrointestinal bleeding. Aspirin preventive therapy is not recommended for younger patients or those 80 and older.

116. C: If an advanced practice registered nurse is assessing cholesterol levels, the value that is of most concern is triglycerides, which is elevated and reflects carbohydrate intake.

LDL cholesterol	<100: 100-129: 130-159: 160-189: ≥190:	Optimal Near optimal Borderline high High Very high
Total cholesterol	<200 200-239 ≥240	Optimal Borderline high High
HDL cholesterol	<40 ≥60	Low High (optimal)
Triglycerides	<150 150-199 200-499 ≥500	Normal Borderline-high High Very high

117. D: The advanced practice registered nurse's prescriptive authority is regulated by the state's nurse practice act, so prescriptive authority may vary from one state to another. However, if the prescriptive authority includes prescription of controlled substances, the APRN must apply for Drug Enforcement Agency (DEA) registration. Some states allow the APRN to diagnose and treat without supervision, but other states require that the APRN work with complete or partial physician supervision.

118. D: This score indicates severe disease, ischemia.

ABI scoring	
>1.4	Abnormally high, may indicate calcification of vessel wall.
1.0-1.4	Normal reading, asymptomatic.
0.9-1.0	Low, but acceptable unless there are other indications of PAD.
0.8-0.9	Likely some arterial disease is present.
≤0.6-0.8	Borderline perfusion.
0.5-0.8	Moderate arterial disease.
<0.5	Severe arterial disease.

119. A: If a patient is following the Senokot S® protocol for cancer-associated constipation, on the first day the patient should take 2 tablets at bedtime with increasing doses for 3 days if no results:

- 2 tablets BID
- 3-4 tablets BID or TID
- If no BM by the next day, rule out impaction and take bisacodyl 2-3 tablets TID and/or at bedtime. If impacted, resolve. If not impacted, give additional laxatives, such as lactulose (45-60 mL), magnesium citrate (8 oz.), bisacodyl suppository, or Fleet enema.

If patient has less than one bowel movement per day, the protocol should be stepped up, but if more than 2 per day, the protocol should be stepped back.

120. A: If one intervention out of many possibilities is implemented to solve a problem and data analysis shows the intervention is not effective, then the best solution is to return to the list of possible solutions and to choose a different one to implement on a trial basis. It should not be necessary to completely begin the process again, and failure should be recognized and dealt with effectively rather than prolonged. Full implementation should not be carried out if results of the trial implementation were negative.

121. C: If a patient hospitalized with renal disease develops pneumonia, in order to be categorized as 'hospital-acquired pneumonia" (HAP), the pneumonia must not be present on admission and must occur 48 hours or more after admission. If the pneumonia occurs prior to that time, the infection was likely contracted prior to admission. Healthcare-associated pneumonia occurs within 90 days of hospitalization or 30 days of other contact with healthcare providers, such as for wound care or chemotherapy.

122. A: If a patient with chronic hypertension is beginning the DASH (dietary approaches to stop hypertension diet), the person should eat 6 or fewer ounces of lean meat, poultry, or fish daily. Total fat 27%, Saturated fat 6%, protein 18%, and carbohydrates 55%.

Food group	**Daily servings**
Grains (whole grains preferred)	6-8
Vegetables and fruits	4-5 each
Fat-free or low-fat milk/milk products	2-3
Lean meat, poultry, fish	≤6 (serving = 1 ounce)
Nuts, seeds, legumes	4-5 per week

Food group	Daily servings
Fats and oils	2-3
Sweets and added sugars	≤5 per week

123. C: The 3 basic types of failures in an organization are:

- Skill-based: Slips occur when the individual has the correct intent but does not carry out an action (such as intended mistakenly using the wrong piece of equipment). Mistakes occur when the individual has an incorrect intention that leads to incorrect action.
- Rules-based: The individual incorrectly applies a rule, applies a bad or wrong rule, or fails to apply the correct rule (injury because of failing to assess safety before assisting a patient).
- Knowledge-based: Knowledge is inadequate for situation.

124. D: If a patient hospitalized for renal failure is frightened she may die and upset and tells the advanced practice registered nurse that her biggest regret is having to give a child up for adoption when she was young, the APRN should keep this information confidential. Patients often divulge information, especially when under stress, that is unrelated to their medical condition and will not affect treatment. In those cases, the information should not be shared although it may be appropriate to share that the patient is upset about personal issues.

125. C: If, when interviewing a patient, the advanced practice registered nurse notes that the patient is tapping his foot, moving his legs, and fidgeting with his clothes, the APRN recognizes that these actions may indicate nervousness. Patients may also twist their hair or frequently change position. Some patients may rub their hands together as a comforting measure. The APRN should carefully observe the patient's gestures, posture, eye contact, and distance as these can help to assess how the patient is feeling.

126. D: If the advanced practice registered nurse must visit a number of different patients administering medications and treatments, the APRN should try to document as soon as possible after each administration or treatment to ensure that nothing is forgotten and to avoid the risk of duplicated treatments. Routine care, such as assisting patients to bathe or walk, can be charted every 1-2 hours. Documenting should not be done only at the end of the shift.

127. B: The patient that puts a patient at increased risk and may interfere with recovery and/or compliance is vulnerability. Factors that may make the patient more vulnerable include fear, lack of support, chronic illness, anxiety, and lack of adequate information about disease, treatment options, and/or resources. Patients who are homeless, elderly, or mentally ill are also vulnerable. Poverty and lack of adequate insurance are important factors in vulnerability.

128. A: If a patient has Broca's aphasia and can understand but cannot produce language, the advanced practice registered nurse can provide the patient with picture charts so that patient can point to what is needed. Pictures may include glasses of water, food, fruit, toilet, shower, linen, clothes. The FACES pain scale may be helpful in allowing the patient to indicate the level of pain. Patients may also understand gestures and may be able to learn some hand signs to indicate needs.

129. B: If a patient who has had frequent hospitalizations for heart disease develops severe diarrhea associated with *Clostridioides difficile* infection, both standard and contact precautions should be used for the duration of the disorder because the spores are highly infective and resistant to most disinfectant processes. Careful handwashing with soap and water is essential as well because outbreaks can occur from spores carried on healthcare workers clothes and/or hands.

130. A: When conducting a history under Medicare documentation guidelines, the elements that must be covered include:

- Problem-focused: Chief complaint (CC) and brief history of present illness (HPI) with 1-3 elements.
- Expanded problem-focused: CC, brief HPI, and problem pertinent review of systems (ROS).
- Detailed: CC, extended HPI (≥4 elements), extended ROS, and pertinent past, family and/or social history (PFSH).
- Comprehensive: CC, extended HIP, complete ROS, and complete PFSH.

Each type of history has a separate billing code.

131. C: If the advanced care registered nurse is carrying out a needs assessment to determine what needs in palliative and hospice care are unmet, the first step is to identify the population to be assessed. Subsequent steps include:

- Determine the information needed.
- Select data collection methods.
- Develop tools, such as questionnaires or interview questions, and data collection procedures.
- Train data collectors.
- Select a representative sample of the whole aggregate if necessary.
- Conduct the needs assessment.
- Analyze the data and identify needs.

132. C: If when conducting the history and physical examination of a patient, the advanced practice registered nurse leans forward when the patient is talking and nods the head, occasionally making comments and asking questions for clarification, this is an example of active listening. As part of active listening, the APRN needs to direct attention to the patient and observe nonverbal behaviors, such as the patient's posture, eye contact, facial expression, and tone of voice.

133. A: If a stroke patient's family has elected to place the patient, who is no longer able to make decisions, on hospice care, the 2 criteria that must be met include (1) Palliative Performance Scale (PPS) equal to or less than 40% and (2) poor nutritional status/inability to maintain adequate food and fluid intake as demonstrated by one or more of the following:

- Loss of 10% or greater amount of weight in the previous 6 months
- Loss of 7.5% of greater amount of weight in the previous 3 months
- Serum albumin less than 2.5 g/dL
- Current evidence of pulmonary aspiration that is not responsive to speech therapy interventions.

134. B: If a hospice patient who is no longer responsive has developed coolness in the extremities, progressing from distal to proximal, this usually means that death will occur within 2-3 hours. This is an indication that circulation is beginning to shut down and blood is being shunted to the internal organs, and blood pressure and pulse are beginning to decrease. The family should be advised that death is imminent and family members called if they are not present and wish to be.

135. C: The most common cause of hiccups in palliative and hospice care patient is gastric distention; therefore, initial treatment often includes simethicone or metoclopramide. Various non-pharmacological methods, such as breath holding, may provide some relief. Muscle relaxants, such as baclofen, may benefit some patients. If the patient receives no relief from more conservative treatment and the hiccups are causing pain or marked distress, then more aggressive treatments, such as anticonvulsants or antipsychotic drugs, may be tried, but the patient may develop adverse effects, such as drowsiness.

136. D: If a patient with systemic lupus erythematosus has had some serious complications in the past few years, but recently the patient's disease has been stable but the patient appears more hyperactive than usual and has begun to complain of a wide variety of complaints, the advanced practice registered nurse should assess the patient for depression. When complaints involve multiple systems and no discernible pattern and the patients exhibits changes in behavior, even though the patient does not appear sad or depressed, the patient may be exhibiting atypical signs of depression.

137. B: The advanced practice registered nurse should advise a patient to avoid taking St. John's wort when taking immunosuppressant drugs. St. John's wort is commonly used to treat depression and anxiety; however, it may interact with many different drugs, so if patients indicate an interest in taking the herbal preparation, the APRN should carefully review the patient's list of drugs. St. John's wort should also not be taken with antibiotics, birth control pills, antidepressants, warfarin, anticonvulsants, MAO inhibitors, antiviral medications, and migraine drugs.

138. C: When using music therapy along with relaxation exercises to reduce a patient's anxiety, the best type of music is the patient's preference. An older adult, for example, might find orchestral or classical music soothing while a younger patient may make a very different choice. People may want to listen to music that reflects their ethnic or cultural background. There is no wrong choice although fast and loud music tends to be more stimulating than slower and quieter music.

139. A: A COPD patient may need continuous oxygen to relieve dyspnea when the PaO_2 and oxygen saturation reach $PaO_2 \leq 50$ mmHg or oxygen saturation ≤85% at rest. If the patient has other signs and symptoms, such as cor pulmonale, peripheral edema, pulmonary hypertension, or hematocrit greater than 56%, then the patient may need continuous oxygen with PaO_2 up to 59 mmHg and oxygen saturation to 89%. The critical value for PaO_2 is 40 mmHg.

140. C: If a patient who did not seek medical care for years after developing a breast lesion has a large fungating lesion that has enveloped the left breast with copious amounts of foul-smelling drainage, metronidazole in gel or solution form may help to control infection and decrease odor. The lesion may be irrigated with the solution to cleanse it and then metronidazole gel applied and absorbent dressings. Hydrogen peroxide may be irritating to the tissue, and Dakin's solution has a strong odor. People have tried various other things, such as yogurt and buttermilk, but with little effectiveness.

141. D: The diagnosis that puts patients most at risk for the development of anorexia/cachexia syndrome is cancer. While patients with some types of cancer, such as cancers that make swallowing difficult, may derive some benefit from enteral or parenteral feedings, especially if needed for a limited period of time, cancer patients in general show little benefit long-term from these nutritional approaches. Up to 86% of patients with end-stage cancer develop anorexia/cachexia syndrome.

142. A: If a hospice patient complains of frequent nausea and vomiting, the advanced practice registered nurse should begin treatment by assessing the pattern of nausea and vomiting. For example, the APRN should determine if the nausea and vomiting occur at the same times, before or after meals, and before or after medications or activities. The APRN should try to identify triggers, such as brushing the teeth or smelling certain odors. If a cause and effect relationship can be identified, then controlling the nausea and vomiting is easier.

143. C: If a patient is following the Senokot S® protocol for cancer-associated constipation and has not had a bowel movement after the first day, on the second day the patient should take 3-4 tablets BID. If no BM by the next day, rule out impaction and take bisacodyl 2-3 tablets TID and/or at bedtime. If impacted, resolve. If not impacted, give additional laxatives, such as lactulose (45-60 mL), magnesium citrate (8 oz.), bisacodyl suppository, or Fleet enema. If patient has less than one bowel movement per day, the protocol should be stepped up, but if more than 2 per day, the protocol should be stepped back.

144. C: A 72-year-old patient with chronic heart disease and blood readings that have stabilized at about 150/94 would be categorized as having stage 1 hypertension.

- Normal BP: <120/80
- Prehypertension: 120-130/80-89 mmHg
- Stage 1 hypertension: 140-159/90-99 mmHg
- Stage 2 hypertension: ≥160/100

Systolic BP over 140 mmHg poses a greater threat to health than elevated diastolic pressure.

145. B: If a male patient has urinary incontinence that is characterized by small leakages of urine, difficulty initiating flow (requiring the patient to strain to urinate), and post-urination dribbling of urine as well as frequency, these signs and symptoms are consistent with overflow incontinence. The incontinence usually results from an over-distended bladder and inability to completely empty the bladder during urination. Overflow incontinence is most common in male patients and often results from prostatic hypertrophy.

146. A: If a palliative care patient recently suffered a stroke and has regained strength but has residual weakness, expressive aphasia, difficulty with math, and short-term memory loss, and exhibits slow cautious behavior and needs repeated instructions to carry out tasks, the part of the brain affected by the stroke is the left hemisphere. The weakness is on the right side and the patient may have a right visual field deficit, making it difficult for the patient to judge distance.

147. D: A patient with hypertension, heart disease, and obstructive sleep apnea should use the CPAP machine whenever sleeping—every night and for all naps. With obstructive sleep apnea, passive collapse of the pharynx occurs during sleep, resulting in apneic periods that may last up to 60 seconds and may occur up to 30 times a night. These apneic periods correspond to bradydysrhythmia during apnea and tachydysrhythmia when breathing resumes, stressing the heart. Patient often exhibit daytime symptoms that include somnolence, headache, depression, personality changes, and impotence.

148. C: If a patient with Alzheimer's disease becomes increasingly agitated in the evening and gets in and out of bed at night and wanders about the house and empties the drawers in her room repeated, the patient is experiencing sundowner's syndrome. This is a common sign of increasing dementia. If the patient takes frequent or long naps during the daytime, then the caregiver should try to reduce daytime sleeping to encourage longer sleep periods at night.

149. A: Total parenteral nutrition (TPN) is an intravenous hypertonic solution containing glucose, fat emulsion, protein, minerals, and vitamins. If a patient receiving TPN because of severe dysphagia exhibits signs of azotemia with evidence of dehydration (dry mucous membranes, decreased skin turgor) as well as increased BUN and urine specific gravity, management includes decreasing amino acids in the TPN formula or changing to NephrAmine® solution.

150. B: When instructing a patient with chronic constipation in bowel retraining, the advanced practice registered nurse advised the patient that the best time to schedule defecation is usually 20-30 minutes after a meal because eating stimulates the gastrocolic reflex and this propels fecal material through the colon. A stimulus (suppository, enema, digital stimulation, hot drink) may be needed initially to promote defecation but the goal is to decrease such use over time.

151. D: Protein-calorie malnutrition (marasmus) results from inadequate intake of both protein and calories and is common in patients with chronic illness and is characterized by gradual weight loss with intact visceral protein but loss of skeletal muscle mass; therefore, patients are often very thin or emaciated in appearance. Symptoms include decreased basal metabolism, lack of subcutaneous fat, tissue turgor, bradycardia, and hypothermia. Protein malnutrition (kwashiorkor) is characterized by rapid loss of visceral protein while skeletal muscle mass is retained, making it more difficult to detect.

152. C: If the average person requires about 0.8 g of protein per kilogram daily, a person with a wound should have 1.25-2.0 g/kg daily in order to promote healing. Other daily needs needed for healing include:

- Vitamin A: 1600-2000 retinal equivalents
- Vitamin C: 100-1000 mg
- Zinc: 15-30 mg
- B vitamins: 200% of RDA
- Iron: 20-30 mg

153. B: If a patient is admitted to the unit with a 7 X 10 cm coccygeal pressure ulcer and, on examination, the advanced care registered nurse notes that the exudate is green and a strong foul sweet-smelling odor is present, the most likely infective agent is *pseudomonas*. *Pseudomonas* infections are aggressive and are common in hospitalized patients whose immune systems are depressed. *Pseudomonas* favors a moist environment. Treatment includes antibiotics although organisms are becoming increasingly resistant to treatment.

154. C: If an older patient who suffered a fall from a hospital bed, resulting in a in a head injury and scalp laceration, has a Glasgow Coma Score of 10, this indicates a moderate head injury. The GCS measures three parameters—best eye response, best verbal response, and best motor response—with a total possible score that ranges from 3 to 15 Scores:

- 3 to 8: Coma
- ≤8: Severe head injury
- 9 to 12: Moderate head injury
- 13 to 15: Mild head injury

155. A: If a patient with cirrhosis of the liver has portal hypertension with ascites, the patient is especially at risk for hemorrhage from esophageal varices. Portal hypertension results from obstructed blood flow increasing blood pressure throughout the portal venous system, preventing the liver from filtering blood and causing the development of collateral blood vessels that return unfiltered blood to the systemic circulation. This causes increased serum aldosterone level, which in turn causes sodium and fluid retention in the kidneys, resulting in hypervolemia, ascites, and esophageal varices.

156. A: The following blood gas values indicate respiratory acidosis:

- H: 7.26 (Normal value 7.35-7.45)
- $PaCO_2$: 57 mmHg (Normal value 35-45 mmHg)
- PaO_2: 53 mmHg (Normal value ≥80 mmHg)
- HCO_3: 22 mEq/L (Normal value 22-26 mEq/L)
- Oxygen saturation: 84% (Normal value ≥95%)

The respiratory acidosis is uncompensated because the HCO_3 value increases with compensation. Respiratory acidosis occurs when ventilation of the alveoli is inadequate and gaseous exchange is impaired, resulting in $PaCO_2$ levels increasing and PaO_2 levels decreasing.

157. D: If a 72-year-old female underwent a CABG because of severe chronic coronary artery disease and has been recovering well, but on the second post-operative day the patient has an acute sudden change in consciousness characterized by language disturbance, disorientation, confusion, and visual hallucinations, and the signs and symptoms are fluctuating, the most likely cause is delirium. Up to 40% of older hospitalized patients and 80% of patient with terminal illness develop delirium. Treatment includes trazadone, lorazepam, or haloperidol.

158. B: If a patient who suffers from chronic alcoholism and amphetamine use has complaints of eye pain and, on examination, the advanced practice registered nurse notes that the patient seems confused and is ataxic when ambulating, these signs and symptoms suggest the triad of symptoms common to Wernicke's encephalopathy. This condition results from brain damage to the thalamus and hypothalamus because of inadequate thiamine (B1). Treatment includes IV fluids and thiamine injections to prevent progression to Wernicke-Korsakoff syndrome.

159. C: If the advanced practice registered nurse notes that patients never seem to have adequate pain relief when opioids are administered by another nurse, and this same nurse frequently offers to work double shifts and take on other patients, the APRN should suspect that the nurse is diverting drugs for personal use. The APRN should immediately report the concerns to administration but should not confront the nurse directly or alert the nurse to the concerns.

160. A: If the advanced practice registered nurse is working with and supervising the clinical practice of a graduate student preparing to enter the field for a semester of study and providing feedback that helps to determine the student's grade, the APRN is serving in the role of preceptor. The APRN should include the student in all APRN activities and help the student to understand his/her role. Preceptoring is usually a time-limited (one semester) arrangement.

161. B: The following situations indicate the need for a patient/family conference:

- Family members have unrealistic expectations of patient.
- Patient and family have conflicts regarding patient needs or care.
- Patient and family are unable to communicate effectively.
- Patient and/or family seem confused about patient's condition.

In some cases, a spiritual adviser may be present during the conference or other team members (such as a nutritionist or occupational therapist), depending on the situation.

162. C: If patient has advanced pancreatic cancer that has metastasized to the bowel and liver and asks if having chemotherapy will prolong her life indefinitely, the healthcare providers agrees that this is possible even though the healthcare provider knows that chemotherapy usually only prolongs life a few months, the ethical principle that the healthcare provider has violated is veracity. The healthcare provider is obligated to not only tell the truth but to avoid making misleading statements or evading the truth.

163. D: If a patient is dying, in addition to analgesics, medications that are usually administered as long as possible include antipyretics and antiemetics because they help to maintain patient comfort. Medications that are usually discontinued a few days before death include antihypertensives, diuretics, hormones, antibiotics, hypoglycemic agents, antidysrhythmics, and laxatives. Corticosteroids should be tapered rather than abruptly discontinued.

164. B: If a patient's family member administers an intentional overdose of a prescription opioid without the physician's knowledge (although the physician ordered the drug) in order to bring about a patient's death because the patient asks the family member to do so, this would be classified as homicide. Despite the best intentions, it is not legal to purposely put a patient to death. In states in which physician-assisted is legal, the patient must follow a legal procedure.

165. A: The advanced practice registered nurse should first consider forming a professional development plan during the novice stage of clinical competence, which is at the beginning of the APRN's career when the APRN has little experience. The APRN should always have a goal in mind and take steps to maintain currency in knowledge through study, practice, and research. Benner's stages of clinical competence include novice, advanced beginner, competent, proficient, and expert.

166. D: If the advanced care registered nurse is serving as a consultant to a home health agency regarding palliative care and when asked to carry out a consultation for a patient, the APRN's first step should be to assess the appropriateness of the request, obtaining data to review. Based on data and observation/evaluation, the APRN should make recommendations for interventions and document findings and recommendations. The APRN should obtain feedback regarding the effectiveness of interventions.

167. D: If a patient with persistent urinary frequency associated with overactive bladder has been treated with oral oxybutynin and tolterodine but both oral medications in regular and extended release forms resulted in severe dry mouth, the advanced practice registered nurse should recommend switching to transdermal patches (such as oxybutynin TDS). The transdermal patches usually do not result in dry mouth and provide better bioavailability of the drug although they may cause some local skin irritation.

168. B: If, as a team leader, the advanced practice registered nurse presents a problem to the team and asks members to arrive at a solution although the APRN usually makes the final decision, this type of leadership is classified as democratic. This democratic approach may, in some cases, delay decision-making because of the need to include others and leave time for discussion, but team members are often more committed to decisions because their opinions have been considered.

169. A: If a 28-year-old patient is not able to work, her husband makes minimum wage, and the patient has no insurance and requires expensive treatment, the resource that is most appropriate for the patient is Medicaid, a combined federal and state welfare program authorized by Title XIX of the Social Security Act to assist people with low income with payment for medical care. Each state administers its own Medicaid program, so eligibility criteria and funding may vary.

170. D: If an 80-year-old patient has developed constant dribbling of urine and the patient is no longer ambulatory and spends most of his time in bed or in a chair, the most appropriate option is likely an external condom catheter. Indwelling catheters pose the risk of infection, and may become accidentally pulled out, causing trauma. Adult containment briefs must be changed frequently to avoid skin irritation and may feel uncomfortable to the patient.

171. C: If a patient has a stage III pressure ulcer, a contraindication for treatment with negative pressure wound therapy (NPWT) is exposed vessels because the suction may cause further trauma and bleeding. Other contraindications include malignant wounds and osteomyelitis. NPWT devices provide suction at 75-125 pounds of pressure. The dressing is usually removed, wound examined, and dressing reapplied 2-3 times weekly. NPWT is used after debridement and is especially effective for wounds with large amounts of exudate and those that are slow healing.

172. B: If a patient is at risk for venous ulcers because of peripheral venous insufficiency, the class of compression stocking that is most appropriate is class II. Stocking:

- Class I: 20-30 mmHg, used to provide support for varicose veins
- Class II: 30-40 mmHg, used to prevent venous ulcers
- Class III: 40-50 mmHg, used for treatment of refractory venous ulcers and to control lymphedema
- Class IV: 50-60 mmHg, used for treatment of severe lymphedema

173. A: After application of eutectic mixture of local anesthetic (EMLA) cream (lidocaine 2.5% and prilocaine 2.5%) to a wound prior to debridement, the wound should be covered with plastic wrap for at least 60 minutes before the catheter placement to allow time for the tissue to numb. Some patients may develop transient local reactions, such as blanching, erythema, pruritus, and rash. Systemic reactions are rare. A one-gram dosage is 3.8 cm in length and 5 mm in width.

174. B: If a patient's treatment has not been covered by Medicare and the patient wants to file an appeal, the first level of appeals is a redetermination. The five levels of appeals include:

1. Redetermination: Claims reviewed by a different Medicare Administrative Contractor (MAC).
2. Reconsideration: Case reconsidered by a Qualified Independent Contractor (QIC).
3. Hearing: Case reviewed at a hearing before an Administrative Law Judge (ALJ)
4. Review: Medicare Appeals Council reviews the case.
5. Judicial review: Case goes to the US District Court.

175. D: If an adolescent patient hospitalized for leukemia has been unfailingly cheerful, avoids talking about the disease, and is making plans for an upcoming dance at school even though the patient is severely immunocompromised, the defense mechanism that the patient is likely using to help cope is suppression.

Suppression	**Trying to forget**	**Consciously choosing not to deal with issues.**
Repression	Forgetting.	Unconsciously failing to recall traumatic incidents/feelings.
Sublimation	Redirecting feelings/impulses	Finding a socially-acceptable way to express feelings/impulses.
Denial	Refusing to believe	Seeking other opinions, changing doctors.

Answer Key and Explanations

Online Resources

Due to our efforts to try to keep this book to a manageable length, we've created a link that will give you access to all of your online resources:

mometrix.com/resources719/achpn

It's Your Moment, Let's Celebrate It!

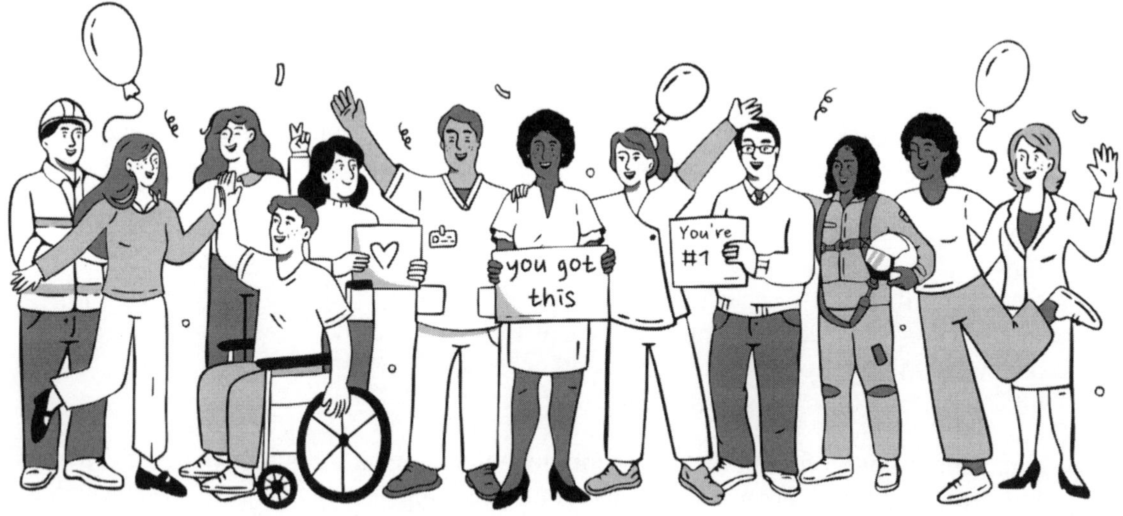

Share your story @mometrixtestpreparation